T0226411

Hallux Abducto Valgus Surgery

Editor

BOB BARAVARIAN

CLINICS IN PODIATRIC MEDICINE AND SURGERY

www.podiatric.theclinics.com

Consulting Editor
THOMAS ZGONIS

April 2014 • Volume 31 • Number 2

ELSEVIER

1600 John F. Kennedy Boulevard • Suite 1800 • Philadelphia, Pennsylvania, 19103-2899

http://www.theclinics.com

CLINICS IN PODIATRIC MEDICINE AND SURGERY Volume 31, Number 2
April 2014 ISSN 0891-8422, ISBN-13: 978-0-323-29012-8

Editor: Jennifer Flynn-Briggs
Developmental Editor: Casey Jackson

Clinics in Podiatric Medicine and Surgery (ISSN 0891-8422) is published quarterly by Elsevier Inc., 360 Park Avenue South, New York, NY 10010-1710. Months of issue are January, April, July, and October. Business and Editorial Offices: 1600 John F. Kennedy Blvd., Ste. 1800, Philadelphia, PA 19103-2899. Customer Service Office: 3251 Riverport Lane, Maryland Heights, MO 63043. Periodicals postage paid at New York, NY and additional mailing offices. Subscription prices are $305.00 per year for US individuals, $450.00 per year for US institutions, $155.00 per year for US students and residents, $370.00 per year for Canadian individuals, $544.00 for Canadian institutions, $435.00 for international individuals, $544.00 per year for international institutions and $220.00 per year for Canadian and foreign students/residents. To receive student/resident rate, orders must be accompanied by name of affiliated institution, date of term, and the *signature* of program/residency coordinator on institution letterhead. Orders will be billed at individual rate until proof of status is received. Foreign air speed delivery is included in all *Clinics* subscription prices. All prices are subject to change without notice. POSTMASTER: Send address changes to *Clinics in Podiatric Medicine and Surgery*, Elsevier Health Sciences Division, Subscription Customer Service, 3251 Riverport Lane, Maryland Heights, MO 63043. **Customer Service: 1-800-654-2452 (US). From outside of the US, call 314-447-8871. Fax: 314-447-8029. E-mail: JournalsCustomerService-usa@elsevier.com (for print support); JournalsOnlineSupport-usa@elsevier.com (for online support).**

Reprints. For copies of 100 or more of articles in this publication, please contact the Commercial Reprints Department, Elsevier Inc., 360 Park Avenue South, New York, NY 10010-1710. Tel.: 212-633-3874; Fax: 212-633-3820; E-mail: reprints@elsevier.com.

Clinics in Podiatric Medicine and Surgery is covered in *MEDLINE/PubMed (Index Medicus)* and *EMBASE/Excerpta Medica*.

Printed and bound by CPI Group (UK) Ltd, Croydon, CR0 4YY

CLINICS IN PODIATRIC MEDICINE AND SURGERY

CONSULTING EDITOR
THOMAS ZGONIS, DPM, FACFAS

Contributors

CONSULTING EDITOR

THOMAS ZGONIS, DPM, FACFAS
Associate Professor, Division of Podiatric Medicine and Surgery, Department of
Orthopaedic Surgery, University of Texas Health Science Center San Antonio,
San Antonio, Texas

EDITOR

BOB BARAVARIAN, DPM
Chief of Podiatric Foot and Ankle Surgery, Santa Monica/UCLA Medical Center and
Orthopedic Hospital, Assistant Clinical Professor, UCLA School of Medicine; Co-Director,
University Foot and Ankle Institute, Los Angeles, California

AUTHORS

BOB BARAVARIAN, DPM
Chief of Podiatric Foot and Ankle Surgery, Santa Monica/UCLA Medical Center
and Orthopedic Hospital, Assistant Clinical Professor, UCLA School of Medicine;
Co-Director, University Foot and Ankle Institute, Los Angeles, California

ROTEM BEN-AD, DPM
Fellow, University Foot and Ankle Institute, Santa Monica, California

MICHAEL BOWEN, DPM
Fellow, Department of Podiatry, Weil Foot and Ankle Institute, Des Plaines, Illinois

PATRICK R. BURNS, DPM, FASPS
Assistant Professor of Orthopaedic Surgery, Director, Podiatric Medicine and Surgery
Residency, University of Pittsburgh Medical Center, Pittsburgh, Pennsylvania

L. MAE CHANDLER, DPM, AACFAS
University Foot and Ankle Institute, Santa Barbara, California

SUZANNE T. HAWSON, PT, MPT, OCS
Physical Therapist, Department of Physical Therapy, University Foot and Ankle Institute,
Valencia, California

J. BRAXTON LITTLE, DPM, FACFAS
Private Practice, University Foot and Ankle Institute, Santa Monica, California

NICHOLAS J. LOWERY, DPM
Chairman, ADA Special Interest Group – Foot Care 2013–2015; Attending Physician,
UPMC Mercy Podiatric Surgical Residency Program, Pittsburgh, Pennsylvania

BRANDON MECHAM, DPM, PGY-3
Podiatric Medicine and Surgery Residency, University of Pittsburgh Medical Center, Pittsburgh, Pennsylvania

JASON MORRIS, DPM, AACFAS
University Foot and Ankle Institute, Santa Monica, California

DAVID RETTEDAL, DPM
First Year Resident, University of Pittsburgh Medical Center Mercy Podiatric Surgical Residency Program, Pittsburgh, Pennsylvania

MICHAEL RYAN, DPM
Private Practice, Arnold, Pennsylvania

LOWELL WEIL Jr, DPM, MBA, FACFAS
President and Fellowship Director, Department of Podiatry, Weil Foot and Ankle Institute, Des Plaines, Illinois; Partner, Foot and Ankle Business Innovations

Contents

Hallux abductovalgus (HAV) is a common but complex deformity. HAV is a combination of deformities and abnormalities. Because HAV is not from a single cause or pathologic process, controversies in description and potential treatments exist. Although many HAV deformities appear similar, no two are the same and thus cannot be treated the same surgically.

The primary indication for an osteotomy of the hallux proximal phalanx to correct hallux abductovalgus (HAV) deformities is increased hallux interphalangeus. The typical osteotomy is the Akin osteotomy or a variation. The Akin is a medial closing wedge osteotomy in the proximal phalanx. An Akin-type osteotomy is usually used as an adjunctive procedure for HAV to correct deformity within the great toe. When first metatarsal procedures and soft tissue balancing are not sufficient for realigning the first metatarsophalangeal joint, an Akin can be useful. A hallux proximal phalanx osteotomy is not indicated as the primary correction for HAV deformities.

An array of distal first metatarsal osteotomies has been described over the decades for the correction of hallux valgus. No one procedure is proficient in correcting all forms and severities of hallux valgus deformities. To optimize results, it is imperative for the surgeon to match a procedure and its modifications to the patient's deformity. The dorsal long arm chevron osteotomy stands at the forefront for correction of mild to moderate hallux abductovalgus. The results with this specific osteotomy are predictable; it allows for early ambulation, and it is easily modified to compensate for the deformity at hand.

The scarf osteotomy has been used and researched extensively for many years for the correction of hallux valgus deformity in both the adolescent and adult populations. It is an inherently stable construct, which allows for early weight bearing and early return to activities of daily living. The scarf procedure has a wide array of surgical indications with great reproducibility and a low complication rate, and it can be performed bilaterally simultaneously, with long-term predictability. Once the scarf procedure is mastered, it is a rewarding and predictable operation for both the surgeon and patient.

Proximal first metatarsal osteotomies have historically been associated with and limited to treatment of severe hallux valgus deformities. These procedures are powerful in deformity correction and overall realignment of first ray function because of their ability to correct closer to the deformity's origin. When considering all factors in bunion correction, they are good options for correction of a wide range of hallux abducto valgus deformities. This article discusses the use of proximal metatarsal osteotomies for correction of hallux valgus deformity, techniques to facilitate optimal outcome, and common complications of these osteotomies.

Fixation options for hallux valgus correction vary. Although some methods are newer and more advanced, even the older techniques are successful in appropriate situations. Kirschner wires and cerclage wiring have their place in proximal phalanx and first metatarsal osteotomies. They are useful for fusion procedures, depending on patient bone quality. Advancements with staple fixation allow the surgeon to apply compression with this device. One of the most stable forms of fixation is the bone screw. By providing a stable construct with good interfragmentary compression, primary bone healing is facilitated. The more recent use of rigid locking plates has allowed for earlier weight bearing following fusion procedures.

First metatarsophalangeal joint arthrodesis is a reliable procedure with predictable outcomes in the treatment of moderate-to-severe hallux valgus with degenerative changes of the joint. It offers better functional outcome compared to arthroplasty with or without prosthesis in appropriate patient populations. Recent studies have shown that with appropriate fixation, early weight bearing may be initiated without an increase in nonunion.

The need for revision hallux valgus surgery is a problem all surgeons encounter. Revision of a failed hallux valgus surgery is often difficult, and very little research exists and few papers have been presented on the topic. Hallux valgus failure has multiple causes, including reoccurrence, avascular necrosis, malunion, nonunion, and hallux varus. These problems can be difficult to address, although some are far more difficult to correct than others. This article details the underlying causes of hallux valgus failure, the workup, and the revision options, with the hope of providing greater education and research on this difficult problem.

The Lapidus procedure as evolved over the last 50 years. What originally was a difficult procedure with poor outcomes has changed to a procedure that allows for ideal realignment of the deformity at its source, improved foot alignment, and minimal to no need for further surgery. The authors now use a weight bearing plate which has improved overall patient care, with a minimized risk of nonunions, and more rapid return to early weight bearing and range of motion. This method has opened up the procedure to more patients, decreased the recovery time, and allowed for early physical therapy, resulting in outstanding patient outcomes.

This article discusses physical therapy considerations after hallux valgus correction. Hallux valgus is a fairly common occurrence, and corrective surgery is an option when conservative measures fail. Symptoms such as pain, swelling, and difficulty walking may persist after surgical correction of bunion deformity that addresses soft tissue and bone structure. Physical therapy is helpful after corrective hallux valgus surgery to address impairments and continued dysfunction and to improve overall patient outcome expectations. This article describes the benefits of a multifaceted physical therapy program after hallux valgus correction.

CLINICS IN PODIATRIC MEDICINE AND SURGERY

RELATED ISSUE

Clinics in Podiatric Medicine and Surgery
July 2013 (Volume 30, Issue 3, Pages A1–A2, 271–460)
Advances in Forefoot Surgery
Charles M. Zelen, *Editor*

DOWNLOAD
Free App!

Review Articles
THE CLINICS

NOW AVAILABLE FOR YOUR iPhone and iPad

Foreword

Hallux Abducto Valgus Surgery

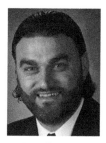

Thomas Zgonis, DPM, FACFAS
Consulting Editor

This edition of *Clinics in Podiatric Medicine and Surgery* focuses on the pathome-chanics and conservative and surgical management of hallux abducto valgus deformities. A variety of topics are well covered, including indications and contraindi-cations of hallux abducto valgus surgical correction at the first metatarsal head, shaft, or base. Equal attention is emphasized at the first metatarsocuneiform arthrodesis procedures for the correction of hallux abducto valgus deformities and proximal phalangeal osteotomies and realignment at the first metatarsophalangeal joint. Last, complications and revisional hallux abducto valgus surgical procedures are discussed in detail.

In this issue, the guest editor, Dr Baravarian, and the invited authors have done an outstanding job in addressing some of the most common procedures used in the surgical correction of the symptomatic hallux abducto valgus deformity. I would like to thank all of the authors and readers for their great contributions and input for *Clinics in Podiatric Medicine and Surgery*.

Thomas Zgonis, DPM, FACFAS
Division of Podiatric Medicine and Surgery
Department of Orthopaedic Surgery
University of Texas Health Science Center San Antonio
7703 Floyd Curl Drive, MSC 7776
San Antonio, TX 78229, USA

E-mail address:
zgonis@uthscsa.edu

Clin Podiatr Med Surg 31 (2014) xi
http://dx.doi.org/10.1016/j.cpm.2014.01.003   **podiatric.theclinics.com**
0891-8422/14/$ – see front matter © 2014 Elsevier Inc. All rights reserved.

Preface

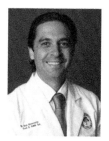

Bob Baravarian, DPM
Editor

Hallux valgus and bunion surgery have evolved dramatically in the past 15 years that I have been practicing. I remember thinking that as long as the metatarsal was positioned over the sesamoids, the foot would heal. I also remember looking sometimes and wondering why things did not work out as well as I thought. Why did the patient scar and get stiff? Why did the bunion come back? Why did a patient have postoperative complications and what caused them?

Throughout my career, I have tried to work toward a better option, a better solution, a more comfortable procedure, and foremost, a faster outcome. What used to take 6 months to heal now commonly takes 6 weeks. What required prolonged periods of no weight-bearing now is done fully weight-bearing. It is under those auspices that I present this latest clinic on hallux valgus correction. My goal is to present the options available, the current rationale, and the most current options.

At University Foot and Ankle Institute in Los Angeles, California, we have been studying bunions and bunion surgery for over 10 years with a single-minded goal of improved and timely outcomes. To that end, we have begun to implement a standardization protocol to our surgeries. We use a special local anesthetic for 72 hours of numbness and pain relief; we use a very light and breathable casting material that is waterproof. We have implemented better rigid fixation to allow weight-bearing without the need for prolonged periods of casting. We also have worked to begin early and often physical therapy to prevent cast disease and get the patient and region moving quickly. This whole process has resulted in outstanding outcomes: less stiffness, less recovery time, and better patient satisfaction.

I want to thank all the authors for their time and contributions. You are all respected in your field and I appreciate you donating your time to this issue. I also want to thank my partners, who I work with every day without which the results and patient outcomes

Clin Podiatr Med Surg 31 (2014) xiii–xiv
http://dx.doi.org/10.1016/j.cpm.2013.12.007
0891-8422/14/$ – see front matter © 2014 Published by Elsevier Inc.

would not continually improve. Finally, I want to thank my family for their understanding and love. All I do, I do for them.

Bob Baravarian, DPM
Department of Surgery
UCLA School of Medicine
Los Angeles, CA, USA

Podiatric Foot and Ankle Surgery
Santa Monica/UCLA Medical Center and Orthopedic Hospital
Santa Monica, CA, USA

University Foot and Ankle Institute
2121 Wilshire Boulevard
Suite 101
Santa Monica, CA 90403, USA

E-mail address:
BBaravarian@mednet.ucla.edu

Biodynamics of Hallux Abductovalgus Etiology and Preoperative Evaluation

Patrick R. Burns, DPM[a],*, Brandon Mecham, DPM[b]

KEYWORDS

- Hallux valgus • Biomechanics • Radiographic evaluation of hallux valgus

KEY POINTS

- Hallux abductovalgus (HAV) is a common but complex deformity.
- HAV is a combination of deformities and abnormalities. Because HAV is not from a single cause or pathologic process, controversies in description and potential treatments exist.
- Although many HAV deformities appear similar, no two are the same and so cannot be treated the same surgically.

INTRODUCTION

Hallux abductovalgus (HAV) is the most common issue of the first metatarsal phalangeal joint (MPJ), affecting 2% to 4% of the population.[1] For many years, the term *bunion* was used to refer to the enlargement seen at the first MPJ, and it was believed to be a simple enlargement or growth of bone. The definition, diagnosis, and treatment, however, may be somewhat confusing. The term *hallux valgus* is now generally accepted. It was introduced by Hueter[2] in 1877 meaning "big toe" and "deviation from the midline." But which deviation was being referenced? Haines and McDougall[3] better described the deformity later. Although the hallux is sometimes purely laterally deviated as hallux valgus, other times it is deviated and rotated in the frontal plane, displacing the sesamoids and causing secondary ligamentous changes (**Fig. 1**). This deformity or pronation of the hallux on the head of the metatarsal adds the abduction to the naming of *hallux abductovalgus*. In reality, HAV is really a combination of

No disclosures.
[a] Department of Orthopaedic Surgery, University of Pittsburgh School of Medicine, University of Pittsburgh Medical Center, 2100 Jane Street, RTMB N7100, Pittsburgh, PA 15203, USA; [b] Podiatric Medicine and Surgery Residency, University of Pittsburgh Medical Center, 2100 Jane Street, RTMB N7100, Pittsburgh, PA 15203, USA
* Corresponding author. Podiatric Medicine and Surgery, University of Pittsburgh Medical Center, 2100 Jane Street, RTMB N7100, Pittsburgh, PA 15203.
E-mail address: burnsp@upmc.edu

Clin Podiatr Med Surg 31 (2014) 197–212
http://dx.doi.org/10.1016/j.cpm.2013.12.002
0891-8422/14/$ – see front matter © 2014 Elsevier Inc. All rights reserved.

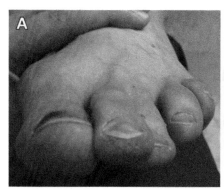 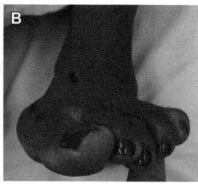

Fig. 1. Clinical examples hallux valgus with mostly transverse plane (*A*) and frontal plane (*B*) components.

deformities and abnormalities. Because no one cause or pathologic process is known, controversies in description and potential treatments exist.

The origins and demographics of HAV are also still debated. Many conditions have been associated with the formation of HAV, including arthritides, metatarsal length, instability, equinus, metatarsus adductus, metatarsal head shape, and pes planus.[1,4,5] Many associations have also been made with age, gender, maternal familial history, occupation, and shoe gear. All of these associations seem to have some support in the literature, although some have stronger evidence than others. In a review of 122 feet, Coughlin and Jones[5] found an 83% familial history, which seems consistent with findings in other literature ranging from 77% to 94%. Good evidence shows that an intrinsic predisposition may be present that may then be activated by other factors, giving rise to HAV. They also found that HAV was present bilaterally in 84% of their population, with 71% having an oval or a round metatarsal head, and 71% having a long first metatarsal. Female sex was much more prevalent at 92%, consistent with other reports quoting 90%.[1,4] Constrictive shoes and occupation seem to play a role at 34%. Other authors have noted populations trending toward closed leather footwear versus barefoot or open sandals, leading to an increased incidence of HAV deformities and complaints.[6] Equinus, increased mobility, metatarsus adductus, and pes planus were not as common, each with a prevalence of less than 15%.

ADULT VERSUS JUVENILE

The age for juvenile HAV is somewhat ambiguous. It is generally accepted to mean skeletal immaturity or open growth plates in the context of HAV (**Fig. 2**). These individuals typically have not had time to form the reactive bone changes to the medial first metatarsal head, and therefore have milder bursa thickening and a relatively small or nonexistent medial eminence. Range of motion (ROM) is not usually affected and no secondary arthritic changes are seen. With time, many of the adult changes occur. The misalignment and subsequent pull of sesamoid ligaments lead to the increased medial eminence and arthritic changes (**Fig. 3**). Although the true incidence is not known, it is reported to range from 20% to 83% by Piggott.[7] Obviously the deformity is influenced by the type of practice, but among the typical demographic seen by the general foot and ankle surgeon, approximately 80% will be adult.[4,5]

For most of these deformities, unless significant pain or deformity exists, nonsurgical management is generally accepted until skeletal maturity occurs in order to limit

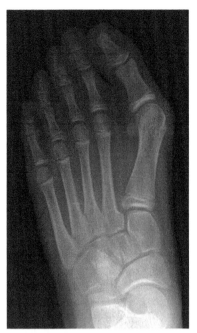

Fig. 2. Radiographic example of HAV in a pediatric patient. Note the deformity in the presence of open growth plates.

continued deformity, allow less chance for recurrence, and provide open access to all types of osteotomies. With open growth plates, potential exists for continued deformity, and therefore incomplete correction or recurrence is a concern. The other issue is obvious limitation to the type of osteotomy available. The growth plate for the first metatarsal is at the proximal end, limiting head or shaft osteotomies that may not address the deformity correctly. The phalangeal osteotomies may also be limited because of the growth plate of the proximal phalanx. The growth plate in theory can be fused laterally, an *epiphysiodesis*, which allows the medial aspect of the metatarsal

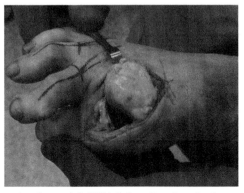

Fig. 3. Operative example of an adult HAV deformity wherein the reactive changes of the first metatarsal head have occurred with time.

to continue growing. This procedure will correct alignment but must have the adequate time to achieve correction, which is difficult to predict. Opening wedge osteotomies of the medial cuneiform have also been described for this abnormality but are not as widely used.[8] Generally, the growth plates reach maturity around 12 to 14 years, and surgeons prefer to wait if possible.

THE FIRST METATARSAL PHALANGEAL JOINT

From an anatomic standpoint, the first metatarsal head is unstable. It has no tendon attachments and is physically small compared with the force placed on it. Because of this, the biodynamics of shape and surrounding structures are even more important for proper function and preventing deformity.

The entire first ray must be included in this section. Although the biodynamics of HAV includes issues ranging from the mobility and relationship of the rearfoot and midfoot, this article concentrates on the first metatarsal cuneiform joint (MCJ) and distal.

Equinus and pes planus have not been shown to directly correlate with the formation of HAV, but many investigators believe they at least have a role.[5] With a predisposition based on inheritance or other issues, such as metatarsal head shape, increased stress on the first MCJ from a rearfoot equinus may lead to drift of the metatarsal. The same holds true for individuals possibly predisposed to instability, such as those with pes planus. These individuals may have an intrinsic laxity in supporting and ligamentous structures in general. If the first MCJ and MPJ are then subjected to certain forces in this state, the hallux may be likely to drift and cause deformity. Unfortunately, instability or hypermobility is not present in every HAV deformity. Although hypermobility seems to be a reasonable explanation and part of some pathologic condition seen, it is present in only 13% of those undergoing correction.[9–11]

THE FIRST METATARSAL CUNEIFORM JOINT

The shape of the first MCJ has been implicated as a common cause of HAV because of its shape.[12–14] The joint approaches 3 cm in depth and has varying shapes. The shape of the actual joint surface may play a role, not just the angle of the joint. In a study of 23 cadaveric specimens in which a total of 37 feet were dissected, Mason[15] identified 3 distinct articular shapes. The first was a unifacet smooth joint across the entire surface. The second was a bifacet joint with 2 distinct articular facets: superior and inferior. The third articular surface subtype identified was a trifacet joint with a large superior, a smaller medial inferior, and a lateral inferior facet. The lateral inferior facet appeared elevated from the other 2. Another finding was a lateral plantar prominence that may be implicated in hypertrophy of the peroneus longus attachment, and a possible part of some forms of HAV.

The first MCJ has no ligamentous attachment to the lateral 4 rays. The second and third rays in particular are very stable, surrounded by not only ligamentous attachments but also a complicated "keystone," or interconnecting pattern of articulations, to provide significant stability. This stability is essential to resist the stress through this part of the foot during gait. The first ray has no such attachments or interlocking articulations, and therefore is inherently unstable compared with the other tarsometatarsal joints. Because the first ray has 2 unstable joints, both at the first MCJ and first MPJ, this leads to the potential for deformity (**Fig. 4**).

These unstable or hypermobile biomechanics can lead to drift of the metatarsal. As the metatarsal drifts medially, the soft tissue imbalance at the first MPJ exacerbates the lateral drift of the hallux. The axis of the long extensor changes and it becomes a deforming force. The lateral capsule is attenuated and the medial structures contract

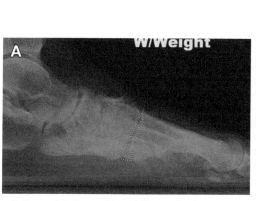

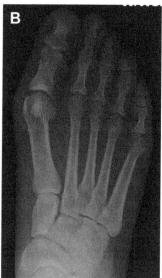

Fig. 4. Potential signs of instability with plantar gapping of the first MCJ (*A*) and a round first metatarsal head (*B*). The (*dotted triangle*) outlines the first metatarsal cuneiform joint, denoting plantar gapping, a potential sign instability.

in response to the change in position. It is a common theory of HAV formation. Lapidus[13] described the classic atavistic joint, a residual shape or trait from evolution that would have allowed a more opposable position for use during climbing or grasping (**Fig. 5**). However, not all HAV has an abnormal first MCJ shape.

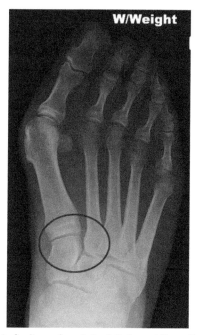

Fig. 5. Typical radiographic finding of an "atavistic" or oblique first MCJ joint axis.

Normal motion at the first MCJ may constitute 41% to 57% of all medial column motion (hypermobile part). No consensus exists on the normal amount of motion at the first MCJ. In 1935, Morton[12] described mobility and its implications as potential causes of many of the pathologic entities of the foot and ankle. These were also implicated by Lapidus[13] and Lake[14] in their theories of HAV formation.

THE SESAMOID APPARATUS

The first MPJ is unique because of its sesamoid bones and surrounding musculature. First, it has 2 sesamoid bones on either side of a cartilage ridge or crista plantar to the first metatarsal head. These sesamoids play a large role in diagnosis and repair of HAV. They function to absorb weight and transmit force during motion through the hallux. They are found within their respective heads of the flexor hallucis brevis tendon, assisting in its mechanical advantage for plantarflexion, while protecting the flexor hallucis longus tendon that courses between. The sesamoids are connected distally to the inferior portion of the base of the proximal phalanx and proximally to the inferior portion of the first metatarsal head proximal to the cartilage. They are connected to each other plantarly by a ligament that envelops the flexor hallucis longus. In conjunction with the suspensory ligaments medial and lateral, this helps form the specialized plantar plate of the first MPJ. The medial and lateral sling-like suspensory ligaments may play a large role in HAV progression and late findings, such as medial eminence formation. They articulate with the first metatarsal head, allowing for increased protection. The sesamoids glide distal and somewhat dorsal during motion of the first MPJ, distributing force and allowing a smooth transition. While standing, the sesamoids tend to be slightly posterior to the metatarsal head, but move distal to protect the exposed head and cartilage during dorsiflexion and gait. The tibial sesamoid tends to be slightly larger and may bear more of the weight, but whether this has clinical implications is unclear.[16] As deformity continues, the crista becomes worn, until the ridge is no longer present to act as a resistance to displacement.

TENDON/MUSCLE OF THE FIRST MPJ

The intrinsic and extrinsic tendons and muscles of the first MPJ can be divided into 4 main groups: dorsal, plantar, medial, and lateral. They all function to enable motion and stability of the joint.

The dorsal muscles include the extensor hallucis longus (EHL) and extensor hallucis brevis (EHB). The EHL provides the power of dorsiflexion, attaching to the dorsal aspect of the base of the distal phalanx. It also gives rise to the extensor hood, enveloping the first MPJ and augmenting the capsule. The EHB inserts on the dorsal aspect of the base of the proximal phalanx just lateral to the EHL, passing by on its way to the distal phalanx. It dorsiflexes the hallux and helps provide local stability. These extensor tendons may play a role in continued or increased HAV, because as the hallux moves lateral, the pull of these tendons present a deforming force. Therefore, the EHB is frequently sacrificed in HAV repair and the EHL sutured back into place more medially to become a more pure dorsiflexor.

Plantar tendons include the flexor hallucis longus (FHL) and flexor hallucis brevis (FHB). The FHB and its importance were discussed earlier, as the sesamoids rest within and help increase the mechanical advantage of plantarflexion. The FHL is the extrinsic plantarflexion workhorse to the hallux. Little further discussion has occurred in the literature about the biodynamic effects of this group.

Medially, the abductor hallucis (AbH) attaches to the medial aspect of the base of the proximal phalanx, and a portion attaches to the tibial sesamoid, contributing to the plantar plate. This structure would aid in overall stability of the first MPJ. From a biodynamic standpoint, it may tend to lengthen or become stretched as HAV progresses. It may not have a direct active role, but rather a more passive one, not being strong enough to resist the forces, thereby allowing the lateral drift. It is not addressed often in HAV repair but may be incorporated into the medial capsulorrhaphy as the soft tissues are balanced.

Laterally, the AbH attaches to the lateral aspect of the base of the proximal phalanx, but also contributes to the plantar plate and its attachment to the fibular sesamoid. The AbH has 2 heads, which may explain part of the pronation mechanism seen in some HAV deformities. It also aids in the stability of the joint, but has also been implicated in the progression of deformity. If it is not an active force pulling the hallux into valgus, it may at least become atrophied or tight with longstanding deformities. For years, addressing this aspect of HAV biodynamics has been one of the mainstays of treatment. Many surgeons still release this tendon as part of soft tissue balancing. That technique has undergone scrutiny recently, with studies showing that the lateral release has no effect on overall outcome, and may even stiffen or decrease ROM.[17–19] Concerns have also been reported about lateral release insulting the blood supply to the head and first MPJ, with possible increases in avascular events.[20] It is true that the first MPJ capsule may become contracted in response to HAV deformities and can be released, but in light of these concerns, a true lateral release of the AbH and surrounding ligaments and tissue may not be beneficial.

HISTORY AND PHYSICAL EXAMINATION

Evaluation of hallux valgus should always begin with taking a thorough history, including the patient's chief complaint. The most common complaint—pain over the medial eminence—is reported in 70% to 75% of this patient population.[5,21] Other common complaints include lesser metatarsalgia and painful, intractable plantar keratosis beneath the second metatarsal head,[21] seen in 48% and 40% of patients with hallux valgus, respectively (**Fig. 6**). Instability and deformity of lesser digits and corns and calluses are common associated complaints. The patient's medical and social histories, including information regarding the patient's activity level, occupation, tobacco use, and reason for choosing surgery, are all highly relevant.

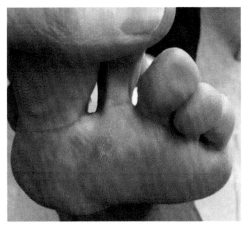

Fig. 6. Clinical findings of second MPJ overload from abnormal first ray biomechanics and HAV.

Physical examination of hallux valgus may begin with a more global approach, including gait analysis and evaluation of the foot with the patient standing and sitting. It is important to examine the patient while weight-bearing and sitting, because the dynamics of HAV can create significant differences in clinical appearance of the deformity while the foot is loaded.[22] The overall size and shape of the deformity of the hallux and lesser digits and any concomitant midfoot or rearfoot misalignment are noted. With the patient in a sitting position, the forefoot-to-rearfoot relationship (eg, varus, valgus, neutral) should be evaluated through loading the lateral column and noting the position of the forefoot relative to the heel (a line perpendicular to the bisection of the heel). ROM of the ankle, subtalar, midtarsal, and first metatarso-phalangeal (MTP) joint are all also evaluated with the patient in a sitting position.

The first MTP joint is evaluated for crepitus or synovitis and is palpated for any specific areas of pain. Passive and active MTP joint ROM should be measured using a goniometer. Manually reducing the deformity while slowly dorsiflexing and plantar-flexing the toe will help determine how much correction may be achieved with surgical correction. Also, the MTP joint ROM will often decrease once the position of the hallux is corrected, suggesting that the articular surface may have adapted to the lateral deviation of the hallux, and that ROM will likely be decreased postoperatively.

Evaluation of the mobility of the first MTC joint is performed by stabilizing the lateral 4 rays in one hand with the first ray held between the thumb and index finger of the other hand. The first metatarsal is then plantarflexed and dorsiflexed, with the remaining metatarsals being held in a stable position (**Fig. 7**). Other clinical signs of hypermobility of the first ray include hyperkeratotic lesions under the lesser metatarsal heads and a functional hallux limitus with decreased dorsiflexion at the MTP joint when the forefoot is loaded.

The lesser MTP joints and digits should be evaluated for instability and deformity, including contractures, hammer toes, mallet toes, and underriding or overriding digits. These deformities are often associated with HAV and may act a significant source of pain; without resolution, patients are likely to experience incomplete pain relief.

A complete neurologic examination should be performed, including testing for vibratory and protective sensations. Often patients may exhibit pain or even a positive Tinel sign with palpation of the dorsomedial cutaneous nerve because of increased local pressures from the medial eminence. Manual muscle-strength testing of all intrinsic and extrinsic musculature of the foot and leg should also be performed.

The vascular evaluation includes a gross examination of the skin and hair patterns, palpation of the dorsalis pedis and posterior tibial pulses, and observation of the capillary refill time in the digits. If these findings are equivocal, then noninvasive vascular

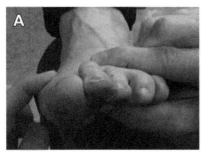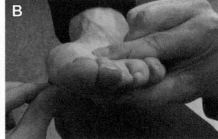

Fig. 7. Clinical examination of the first MCJ placing it through ROM, plantarflexion (A) and dorsiflexion (B) to determine possible hypermobility.

studies should be ordered, including a Doppler examination, segmental pressures (including great toe pressures), and ankle-brachial index.

RADIOGRAPHIC EVALUATION

Radiographic evaluation of the hallux valgus deformity should be performed while the patient is weight-bearing and in their angle and base of gait.[22] Standard views should include anteroposterior, medial oblique, and lateral views. Although many radiographic angles and features are described in the literature, some seem to be of more clinical significance than others. This article focuses on those that are the most clinically relevant.

THE 1–2 INTERMETATARSAL ANGLE

This angle is visualized on an anteroposterior weight-bearing view, with the reference lines being the bisection of the first and second metatarsals.[23] The angle created between these lines forms the 1–2 intermetatarsal angle (**Fig. 8**). This angle is typically used for overall classification of HAV, with the normal value being 0° to 8°, mild deformity characterized as 9° to 12°, moderate deformity as 13° to 16°, and severe deformity as greater than 16°.[1,24] This 1–2 angle for many is the starting point. This basic stratification for years has been used to determine the location of the metatarsal osteotomy. The smaller or mild deformities may be more conducive to a head osteotomy, whereas the larger or severe deformities require a base procedure to more accurately correct the position and therefore biodynamics of the ray.

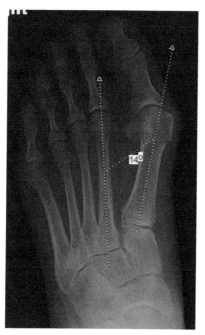

Fig. 8. Radiographic evaluation of first intermetatarsal angle.

HALLUX VALGUS (ABDUCTUS) ANGLE

The hallux valgus angle is measured on an anteroposterior radiograph through comparing the bisections of the first metatarsal and proximal phalanx of the hallux (**Fig. 9**A). Normal values are traditionally 0° to 16°.[24] This angle represents the lateral deviation of the hallux on the first metatarsal, and is by definition increased in HAV.

HALLUX INTERPHALANGEAL ANGLE

On the anteroposterior weight-bearing view, the angle formed by the bisection of the proximal and distal phalanges of the hallux is known as the *hallux interphalangeal angle* (HIA).[4] An angle of less than 9° is typically considered within the normal range (see **Fig. 9**B). It has been noted by multiple authors that an increased HIA has been associated with hallux rigidus, whereas lower HIA seems to be associated with hallux valgus. The prevailing theory is that patients with hallux valgus have less resistance to transverse plane deformity, and thus a decreased HIA.

PROXIMAL ARTICULAR SET ANGLE

Measured on the anteroposterior weight-bearing study, the proximal articular set angle, also known as *distal metatarsal articular angle*, compares a line perpendicular to that created by connecting the points at the most medial and lateral extents of the articular surface of the first metatarsal head with the bisection of the first meta-tarsal.[4] It is useful in evaluating the relationship between the articular surface and longitudinal axis of the first metatarsal (**Fig. 10**). Less than 8° is typically regarded as within the normal range.[25] This angle has some potential issues. The cartilage cannot be visualized, and therefore bone landmarks are used to approximate its location. Because of this, the deformity may be overestimated or underestimated, and may need to be reevaluated during surgery.[26]

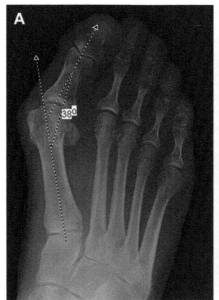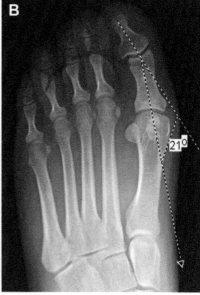

Fig. 9. Radiographic evaluation of HAV (*A*) angle and HIA (*B*) angle.

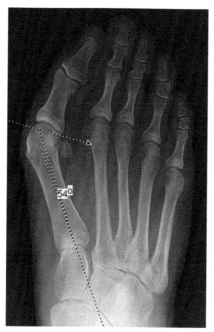

Fig. 10. Radiographic evaluation of proximal articular set angle or distal metatarsal articular angle.

MTP JOINT CONGRUITY AND SHAPE

On the anteroposterior radiograph, the most medial and lateral portions of the articular surface of the metatarsal head and that of the base of the proximal phalanx help determine the congruity of the MTP joint.[27] In a congruent joint, these points will remain concentrically apposed. In a subluxed or noncongruent joint, the medial and lateral points of the articular surfaces of the proximal phalanx will migrate laterally when compared with the corresponding points on the metatarsal head. This fact may prove valuable in determining the proper osteotomy. One would not want to perform an osteotomy and take a congruent deformity and make it incongruent.

The shape of the first metatarsal head should also be evaluated (**Fig. 11**). Round metatarsal heads have been implicated in patients with HAV deformities. This unstable shape makes it difficult for the joint to resist deforming forces, causing it to rely more on the surrounding soft tissue. Any other issues in this biodynamic aspect may then predispose to deviation. The converse is also believed to be true. A square shape to a metatarsal head adds inherent strength, and relieves strain from the local soft tissues. Although this configuration may have its own problems, it lends itself to transverse plane stability and would limit the possible progression of HAV.

MEDIAL EMINENCE

The medial eminence is often at the center of the patient's complaint, and is commonly the focus of both pain and footwear intolerance.[5] Radiographically, the size of the eminence is determined by measuring the difference in millimeters between a line parallel to the medial diaphyseal border of the metatarsal and a line perpendicular at the widest extent of the medial eminence.[28] Although typically perceived by the patient to

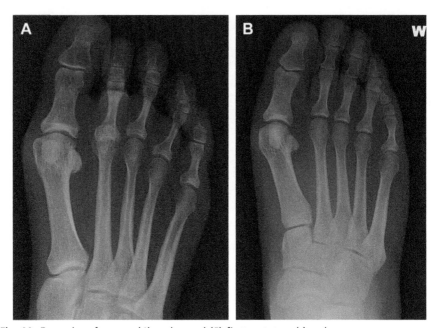

Fig. 11. Examples of square (*A*) and round (*B*) first metatarsal heads.

be the source of the symptoms, the medial eminence for some deformities has been shown to be merely a portion of the metatarsal head exposed by the medially deviating hallux (**Fig. 12**). For others it may be the dorsal medial aspect of the metatarsal when rotated that becomes prominent. Correction of the intermetatarsal angle or rotation of the first ray may remove the perceived bump without requiring resection of the medial metatarsal head.[26] In a study comparing 50 patients with a symptomatic HAV deformity matched versus 50 without, Thordarson and Krewer[28] found no significant difference in the mean thickness of the measured medial eminence.

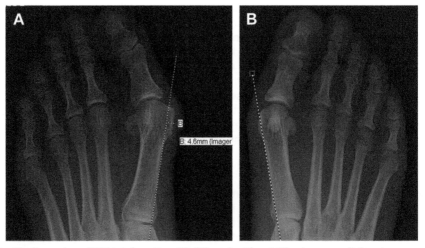

Fig. 12. Examples of HAV deformity with (*A*) and without (*B*) a large medial eminence.

FIRST METATARSAL LENGTH

Length of the first metatarsal can be measured using 2 methods. The first was described by Morton[12] and involves drawing a transverse line from the tip of the first and second metatarsals and measuring the distance between the lines. The second method, proposed by Hardy and Clapham,[24] uses an arc method to measure the difference (**Fig. 13**). Neither method is universally accepted, and no significant correlation ha been noted between metatarsal length and the development of HAV. Measuring metatarsal length may, however, be useful in procedure selection, because most metatarsal osteotomies create shortening. Too much shortening or metatarsal length in general may play a role in lesser metatarsal abnormalities and metatarsalgia issues, but it has not been shown clinically to correlate.[29,30]

TIBIAL SESAMOID POSITION

As the first metatarsal head deviates medially, the soft tissue attachments of the sesamoids, particularly the deep transverse intermetatarsal ligament, anchor the sesamoids in place. This anatomy results in the relative appearance of lateral displacement of both the tibial and fibular sesamoids. This appearance is quantified on the anteroposterior weight-bearing radiograph on a scale of 1 to 7, with a value of 1 assigned when the tibial sesamoid is located medial to the bisection of the first metatarsal, a value of 4 assigned when it is divided by the bisection of the metatarsal, and 7 when it is well lateral to the bisection.[31] Positions 1 through 3 are considered normal (**Fig. 14**). This appearance may serve as an intraoperative landmark to judge reduction of the HAV deformity and effectiveness of the procedure.

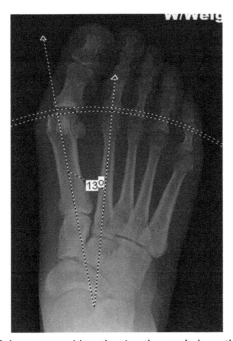

Fig. 13. Evaluation of the metatarsal length using the parabola method.

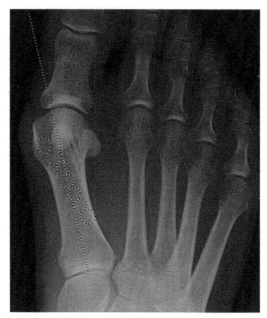

Fig. 14. Radiograph of possible tibial sesamoid positions in HAV deformity.

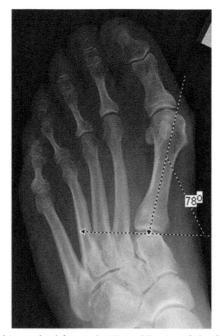

Fig. 15. One radiographic method for evaluating obliquity of the first MCJ.

FIRST METATARSAL CUNEIFORM JOINT ANGLES

The articulation between the base of the first metatarsal and the medial cuneiform plays a critical role in the development of increased 1–2 intermetatarsal angles and the HAV deformity.[3] Vyas and colleagues[32] found that the first metatarsal-cuneiform angle (formed by the long axis of the first metatarsal and the distal articular surface of the medial cuneiform) and the second metatarsal-cuneiform angle (comparing the long axis of the second metatarsal with the distal articular surface of the medial cuneiform) were correlated with increased intermetatarsal angles in patients with juvenile hallux valgus. Because of its anatomic location, a slight deviation at this more-proximal level can lead to greater deformity distally. For this reason, the first MCJ joint is often the center of angular deformity in hallux valgus (**Fig. 15**). Hypermobility at this joint is also commonly thought of as part of the cause of HAV but traditionally has been difficult to evaluate clinically. A radiographic manifestation of this hypermobility is seen on the lateral view as plantar gapping between the metatarsal base and cuneiform.[5] This finding may be one of the only preoperative clues that hypermobility must be addressed, and can help guide procedure selection.

SUMMARY

HAV is a common but complex deformity. Although many instances of HAV seem similar, no 2 are the same, and therefore they cannot be treated the same surgically. Each will have its own nuance. To appreciate how to treat HAV, the foot and ankle surgeon must understand the entire entity, from the anatomy to family history to the biodynamics of the governing joints and tendons, as they all play a role. An a la carte–type approach may be possible, with osteotomies performed based on mobility and radiographic angles but then fine-tuned with adjuncts based on soft tissue and surrounding abnormalities.

REFERENCES

1. Coughlin MJ. Hallux valgus. J Bone Joint Surg Am 1996;78:932–66.
2. Hueter C. Klinik der Gelenkkrankheiten mit Einschluß der Orthopädie. Leipzig (Germany): Vogel; 1877. p. 10–1.
3. Haines RW, McDougall AM. The anatomy of hallux valgus. J Bone Joint Surg Br 1954;36:272–93.
4. Coughlin MJ, Shurnas PS. Hallux rigidus: demographics, etiology, and radiographic assessment. Foot Ankle Int 2003;24:731–43.
5. Coughlin MJ, Jones CP. Hallux valgus: demographics, etiology, and radiographic assessment. Foot Ankle Int 2007;28:759–77.
6. Nork SE, Coughlin RR. How to examine a foot and what to do with a bunion. Prim Care 1996;23(2):293–7.
7. Piggott H. The natural history of hallux valgus in adolescence and early adult life. J Bone Joint Surg 1960;42B:749–60.
8. Jawish R, Assoum H, Saliba E. Opening wedge osteotomy of the first cuneiform for the treatment of hallux valgus. Int Orthop 2010;34(3):361–8.
9. Coughlin MJ, Jones CP. Hallux valgus and first ray hypermobility. A prospective study. J Bone Joint Surg Am 2007;89:1887–98.
10. Coughlin MJ, Smith BW. Hallux valgus and first ray hypermobility. Surgical technique. J Bone Joint Surg Am 2008;90(Suppl Part 2):153–70.
11. Doty JF, Coughlin MJ. Hallux valgus and hypermobility of the first ray: fact and fiction. International Orthopaedics 2013;37:1655–60.

12. Morton DJ. The human foot. New York: Columbia University Press; 1935.
13. Lapidus PW. The author's bunion operation from 1931 to 1959. Clin Orthop 1960; 16:119–35.
14. Lake N. The foot. 3rd edition. London: Bailliere Tindall and Cox; 1945.
15. Mason LW, Tanaka H. The first tarsometatarsal joint and its association with hallux valgus. Bone Joint Res 2012;1(6):99–103.
16. Coughlin MJ. Sesamoids and accessory bones of the foot. In: Mann RA, Coughlin MJ, editors. Surgery of the foot and ankle. 9th edition. St Louis (MO): Mosby; 2007. p. 531–610.
17. Ahn JY, Lee HS, Chun H, et al. Comparison of open lateral release and transarticular lateral release in distal chevron metatarsal osteotomy for hallux correction. Int Orthop 2013;37(9):1781–7.
18. Lee HJ, Chung JW, Chu IT, et al. Comparison of distal chevron osteotomy with and without lateral soft tissue release for the treatment of hallux valgus. Foot Ankle Int 2010;31(4):291–5.
19. Schneider W. Distal soft tissue procedure in hallux valgus surgery: biomechanical background and technique. Int Orthop 2013;37(9):1669–75.
20. Malal JJ, Dunn S, Kumar CS. Blood supply to the first metatarsal head and vessels at risk with a chevron osteotomy. J Bone Joint Surg 2007;89(9):2018–22.
21. Mann RA, Rudicel S, Graves SC. Repair of hallux valgus with a distal soft-tissue procedure and proximal metatarsal osteotomy. A long-term follow-up. J Bone Joint Surg Am 1992;74:124–9.
22. Fuhrmann RA, Layher F, Wetzel WD. Radiographic changes in forefoot geometry with weightbearing. Foot Ankle Int 2003;24:326–31.
23. Coughlin MJ, Saltzman CL, Nunley JA II. Angular measurements in evaluation of hallux valgus deformities: a report of the ad hoc committee of the American Orthopaedic Foot & Ankle Society on angular measurements. Foot Ankle Int 2002;23:68–74.
24. Hardy RH, Clapham JC. Observations on hallux valgus; based on a controlled series. J Bone Joint Surg Br 1951;33:376–91.
25. Richardson EG, Graves SC, McClure JT, et al. First metatarsal head-shaft angle: a method of determination. Foot Ankle Int 1993;14:181–5.
26. Dayton P, Feilmeier M, Kauwe M, et al. Relationship of frontal plane rotation of first metatarsal to proximal set angle and hallux alignment in patients undergoing tarsometatarsal arthrodesis for hallux abducto valgus: a case series and critical review of the literature. J Foot Ankle Surg 2013;52:348–54.
27. Coughlin MJ, Freund E, Roger A. Mann Award. The reliability of angular measurements in hallux valgus deformities. Foot Ankle Int 2001;22:369–79.
28. Thordarson DB, Krewer P. Medial eminence thickness with and without hallux valgus. Foot Ankle Int 2002;23:48–50.
29. Kaipel M, Krapf D, Wyss C. Metatarsal length does not correlate with maximal peak pressure and maximal force. Clin Orthop Relat Res 2011;469:1161–6.
30. Budny AM, Masadeh SB, Lyons MC, et al. The opening base wedge osteotomy and subsequent lengthening of the first metatarsal: an in vitro study. J Foot Ankle Surg 2009;48(6):662–7.
31. Steel MW III, Johnson KA, DeWitz MA, et al. Radiographic measurements of the normal adult foot. Foot Ankle 1980;1:151–8.
32. Vyas S, Conduah A, Vyas N, et al. The role of the first metatarsocuneiform joint in juvenile hallux valgus. J Pediatr Orthop B 2010;19:399–402.

Proximal Phalangeal Osteotomies for Hallux Abductovalgus Deformity

David Rettedal, DPM, Nicholas J. Lowery, DPM*

KEYWORDS

- Hallux abductovalgus • Bunion • Akin osteotomy

KEY POINTS

- Hallux abductovalgus (HAV) is a common deformity treated by foot and ankle specialists.
- In most cases, surgical correction of HAV must address a first metatarsal deformity, and many osteotomies are used for this purpose.
- Proximal phalangeal osteotomies can be a useful adjunct to HAV correction.

INTRODUCTION

Hallux abductovalgus (HAV) is a common deformity treated by foot and ankle specialists. HAV deformity often causes pain with shoes and ambulation that is not amenable to nonoperative treatments, making surgical correction a common end point. In most cases, surgical correction of HAV must address a first metatarsal deformity, and many osteotomies are used for this purpose. In addition to metatarsal correction, however, a deformity inherent to the hallux may exist that, if left unaddressed, could lead to a suboptimal surgical outcome. When this is the case, a proximal phalangeal osteotomy is useful to fully correct the deformity.

Many surgical procedures are used to correct deformity within the hallux, including variations of the Akin osteotomy.[1] Although the original intent of the Akin osteotomy was to correct HAV deformity,[2] the Akin and its variants are now largely used as adjunctive procedures during bunion correction. The Akin osteotomy is best used when deformity is present within the hallux itself, which can be evaluated in the preoperative and perioperative settings. This article discusses variations of phalangeal osteotomies and their value in relation to HAV correction.

PROXIMAL PHALANGEAL OSTEOTOMY

Proximal phalangeal osteotomies in HAV deformities were first described by Akin in 1925.[1,2] The original Akin was described as a medial closing wedge osteotomy

University of Pittsburgh Medical Center Mercy Hospital, 1400 Locust Street, Pittsburgh, PA 15219, USA
* Corresponding author.
E-mail address: lowerynj@upmc.edu

Clin Podiatr Med Surg 31 (2014) 213–220
http://dx.doi.org/10.1016/j.cpm.2013.12.003
0891-8422/14/$ – see front matter © 2014 Elsevier Inc. All rights reserved.

of the hallux proximal phalanx combined with resection of the first metatarsal medial eminence and resection of the medial aspect of the base of the proximal phalanx.[2] This procedure plays a role as an adjunctive procedure in HAV deformities.[3,4] It does not address the increase in intermetatarsal angle or increased proximal articular set angle (PASA), and therefore it should not be used as the primary procedure for HAV. In fact, if used inappropriately as an isolated procedure, an Akin osteotomy could actually worsen the deformity or predispose patients to recurrence.[5]

Although the original orientation for the Akin osteotomy was a medially based closing wedge in the proximal metaphysis of the hallux proximal phalanx,[1,2] the procedure has evolved and now has multiple variations[1] designed to address different levels of deformity or allow for different methods of fixation. Proximal, distal, and oblique Akin osteotomies are now common and are discussed further. Cylindrical variants of the Akin osteotomy are used most commonly for hallux length discrepancies, and although useful for this indication, are not discussed because they do not relate to the correction of HAV deformities.

PREOPERATIVE CLINICAL EVALUATION

Preoperative evaluation begins with clinical and radiographic assessment. Many factors must be considered from a clinical standpoint when evaluating a patient with HAV deformity. The deformity itself is classified as mild, moderate, or severe based on clinical appearance with the patient in stance, and confirmed with angular measurements on weight-bearing radiographs. Range of motion of the first metatarsophalangeal joint is evaluated and measured from a standpoint of quantity and quality. Stability and range of motion of the first ray also requires assessment for hypermobility. When evaluating the hallux itself in isolation, the physician should observe the shape and rotation of the first toe. This important step of the clinical evaluation will help determine the need for a phalangeal osteotomy to assist in the overall correction of the patient's deformity. If the hallux has an interosseous deformity within the proximal phalanx or an intraosseous deformity between its phalanges, this may require attention with surgical correction. If this is the case, the hallux may be in contact with or underlap the second toe, commonly creating concomitant a second ray abnormality.[1]

RADIOGRAPHIC EVALUATION

A thorough radiographic assessment is an important aspect of a preoperative evaluation for HAV deformities. In general, the intermetatarsal 1–2 angle, hallux abductus angle, metatarsus adductus angle, sesamoid position, proximal articular set angle, and first metatarsal length are assessed on anteroposterior radiographs. All of these angles can demonstrate important qualities that relate to the patient's complaint. With regard to the hallux itself, several angles should be evaluated that may indicate the need for phalangeal osteotomy.

Hallux Abductus Angle

The hallux abductus angle represents the angulation between the long axis of the first metatarsal and the longitudinal bisection of the hallucal proximal phalanx.[6] This angle is measured on anteroposterior radiographs, and in normal circumstances measures 15° or less. As this angle increases, the hallux tends to rotate into a valgus malalignment.

Hallux Interphalangeal Angle

The hallux interphalangeal angle is measured on anteroposterior radiographs. This measurement represents the bisection between the proximal phalanx of the hallux and the distal phalanx of the hallux. In normal circumstances, this angle measures 13°.[7] An asymmetry in the articular cartilage of the proximal phalanx or within the distal phalanx itself may cause an increase in this angle.

A longstanding belief exists that an inverse relationship exists between the hallux abductus angle and the hallux interphalangeal angle. When the hallux abductus angle is less than 8°, the hallux interphalangeal angle increases to 16°; inversely, when the hallux abductus angle is greater than 25°, the hallux interphalangeal angle reduces to an average of 9°.[7] The cause or clinical relevance of this relationship remains unclear.

Proximal Articular Set Angle

The PASA is the angulation between the line perpendicular to the first metatarsal articular cartilage and the longitudinal axis of the first metatarsal. In normal circumstances, this angle is 0° to 8°.[6] This angle can increase over time as the hallux drifts laterally with HAV deformity. In orthopedic literature, this angle is commonly referred to as the *distal metatarsal articular angle*. Proximal phalangeal osteotomies are not used to correct PASA. However, this angular deformity, if not properly evaluated, may mislead the treating physician by mimicking a phalangeal deformity.

Distal Articular Set Angle

The distal articular set angle (DASA) is the measurement between the perpendicular to the proximal articular surface of the hallucal proximal phalanx and its longitudinal bisection.[6] This angle represents the orientation between the articular cartilage of the proximal phalangeal base and its longitudinal axis. Normally this angle measures 7° to 9° abducted.[6] When DASA is increased, an interosseous deformity may be seen in the proximal phalanx that will require surgical attention when addressing HAV deformity. Another way to determine this is to measure the medial and lateral sides of the proximal phalanx. If the lateral side is shorter than the medial side, an abduction deformity within the phalanx may be present.

APPLICATION OF PROXIMAL PHALANGEAL OSTEOTOMIES

An HAV deformity that may require the use of an adjunctive hallux osteotomy procedure is one in which a deformity is found within the proximal phalanx itself. The underlying deformity is a hallucal proximal phalanx that has more medial length compared with lateral length, creating a lateral bow within the phalanx, which can be seen clinically and confirmed with radiographs (**Fig. 1**). The basic goal of proximal phalangeal osteotomies for adjunctive hallux valgus correction is therefore to shorten the medial aspect of the proximal phalanx so that the 2 sides have more of a parallel relationship, which results in the toe having a more rectus alignment.[1]

Variations of Proximal Phalangeal Osteotomy

The traditional Akin osteotomy is a medially based closing wedge performed in the proximal metaphysis of the proximal phalanx (**Fig. 2**). It has been used for years for correction of phalangeal and adjunctive HAV deformities; however, for a multitude of reasons, variations of this osteotomy have been created. The type of osteotomy can be influenced by clinical and radiographic parameters described previously, type of fixation or surgeon preference.

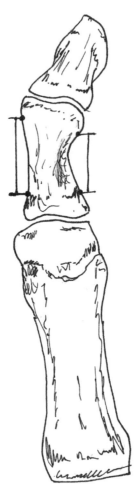

Fig. 1. Example of interosseous phalangeal deformity, with medial side longer than lateral side.

During preoperative evaluation, if an increase in DASA is noted, a traditional Akin osteotomy is best used for correction of this deformity. An increase in DASA indicates a discrepancy between the articular surface of the proximal phalangeal base and the long axis of the proximal phalanx. In this case, the apex of the deformity is in the proximal part of the phalanx and a phalangeal osteotomy near this apex is ideal.

If preoperative evaluation reveals no increase in DASA but an increase in the hallux interphalangeal angle exists, the deformity is intraosseous in nature, located between the proximal and distal phalanges. In this instance, because the deformity is more distal and not solely located in the proximal phalanx, a distal Akin osteotomy may be the preferred procedure. The distal Akin osteotomy is a medially based closing wedge osteotomy but is located in the distal metaphysis of the proximal phalanx **(Fig. 3)**.

Although traditional proximal and distal Akin osteotomies are used today and have clear indications, they also have drawbacks, most notably regarding fixation. For this reason, many surgeons today choose to perform an oblique Akin osteotomy for

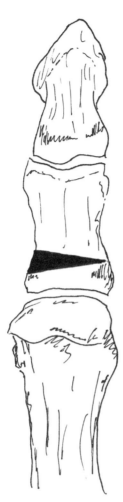

Fig. 2. Traditional proximal akin osteotomy.

enhancement of HAV correction. The oblique Akin osteotomy is again a medially based closing wedge, but it traverses the length of the phalanx in an oblique orientation. It can be oriented from distal-lateral to proximal-medial or vice versa, depending on surgeon preference (**Fig. 4**). The advantages of this osteotomy are the ability to correct phalangeal deformity, regardless of location, and the osteotomy is more amenable to internal fixation, particularly with screws. Disadvantages are the increased exposure needed for performance of the long oblique bone cut, and the delicacy of creating such an osteotomy where the lateral hinge may fracture.

   The author's preference in most circumstances is to use an oblique Akin osteotomy for adjunctive correction of HAV deformity. When performing surgery for HAV deformity, the index procedure is performed first. If, after performance of a metatarsal osteotomy, the first toe is still in valgus alignment, then the decision is made to address the proximal phalangeal deformity. The oblique Akin is oriented from a proximal-lateral apex to a distal-medial closing wedge, and is fixated with a cortical 2.0-mm screw using the lag technique. The complete surgical technique is discussed in the next section.

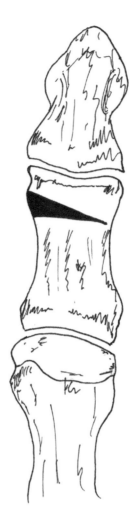

Fig. 3. Distal akin osteotomy.

SURGICAL TECHNIQUE

In most instances, proximal phalangeal osteotomies are performed after a metatarsal osteotomy for HAV. Because of this, the skin incision for the index procedure can be extended longitudinally over the proximal phalanx. After skin incision, soft tissue dissection is carried down to bone, during which the extensor tendons will be encountered and are carefully retracted. Subperiosteal dissection of the proximal phalanx is performed, being mindful of the orientation of the osteotomy.[4] For an oblique Akin osteotomy, greater dissection is required. Once bone is properly exposed, the osteotomy can be planned. The author orients the osteotomy from proximal-lateral to distal-medial. A guide pin can be placed in the proximal-lateral metaphysis of the proximal phalanx at the apex of the osteotomy to protect the lateral hinge when creating the osteotomy. The distal arm of the osteotomy is usually created first, taking care to avoid violating the distal interphalangeal joint. Once the distal arm of the osteotomy is complete (keeping the lateral hinge intact), the proximal arm is then created, removing a small wedge of bone between the 2 cuts. The apical guide pin can be removed,

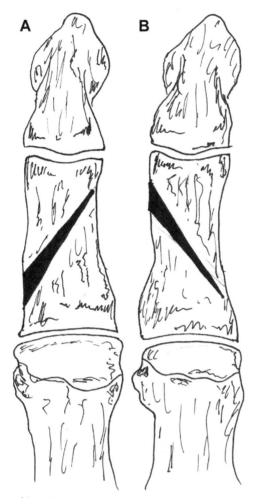

Fig. 4. (*A, B*) Oblique akin osteotomy.

and the osteotomy is gently reduced. If the osteotomy does not easily close, the oscillating saw can then be used to feather the lateral cortex. Once the osteotomy closes, the foot is reassessed, and if the deformity is no longer visible, fixation of the osteotomy is performed. The author prefers to use a 2.0-mm cortical screw oriented perpendicular to the osteotomy, using the lag technique to achieve compression. Any form of fixation can be used, however, including staples, Kirschner wires (K-wires), cerclage wire, or a combination. Once the osteotomy is closed, fixation is stable, and the deformity is properly corrected, the incision is closed in typical fashion. Other variations of the phalangeal osteotomy are described, all of which are aimed at addressing phalangeal deformity.[8–12]

SUMMARY

Proximal phalangeal osteotomies can be useful as an adjunct to HAV correction. Rarely, they are used in isolation for interosseous deformity within the hallux. A diligent preoperative evaluation is necessary to determine both the need for a phalangeal osteotomy and the type of osteotomy. Transverse (proximal and distal) osteotomies are used, depending on the level of deformity. Obliquely oriented phalangeal osteotomies allow for easier use of internal fixation, particularly screw fixation. In addition, staples or K-wires can be used to fixate the osteotomy. If used properly, a phalangeal osteotomy can enhance HAV repair.

ACKNOWLEDGMENTS

The authors would like to thank Carrie Lowery for creating medical illustrations for this article.

REFERENCES

1. Smith T, Moon J. Hallux osteotomies. In: Southerland J, editor. McGlamry's comprehensive textbook of foot and ankle surgery. Philadelphia: Wolters Kluwer Health; 2013. p. 260–78.
2. Akin O. The treatment of hallux valgus: a new operative procedure and its results. Med Sentinel 1925;33:678–9.
3. Mitchell L, Baxter D. A Chevron-Akin double osteotomy for correction of hallux valgus. Foot Ankle 1991;12:7–14.
4. Vanore J. Phalangeal osteotomies. In: Chang T, editor. Master techniques in podiatric surgery: the foot and ankle. Philadelphia: Lippincott Williams and Wilkins; 2005. p. 61–73.
5. Arnold H. The Akin procedure as closing wedge osteotomy for the correction of a hallux valgus interphalangeus deformity. Oper Orthop Traumatol 2008;20(6): 477–83.
6. Sanner WH. Foot Segmental Relationships and Bone Morphology. In: Christman R, editor. Foot and ankle radiology. St Louis: MO Elsevier Science; 2003. p. 272–302.
7. Sorto LA, Balding MG, Weil LS, et al. Hallux abductus interphalangeus: etiology, x-ray evaluation and treatment. J Am Podiatry Assoc 1976;66(6):384.
8. Gerbert J. Textbook of bunion surgery. Philadelphia: WB Saunders; 2001. p. 112–28.
9. Roukis T. Hallux proximal phalanx Akin-Scarf osteotomy. J Am Podiatr Med Assoc 2004;94:70–2.
10. Sabo D. Correction osteotomy of the first phalanx of the great toe (Akin osteotomy). Int Surg 2007;2:66–9.
11. Boberg J, Menn J, Brown W. The distal akin osteotomy: a new approach. J Foot Surg 1991;30(5):431–6.
12. Chacon Y, Fallat L, Dau N, et al. Biomechanical comparison of internal fixation techniques for the Akin osteotomy of the proximal phalanx. J Foot Ankle Surg 2012;51:561–5.

First Metatarsal Head Osteotomies for the Correction of Hallux Abducto Valgus

L. Mae Chandler, DPM, AACFAS

KEYWORDS

- Hallux abducto valgus • Austin bunionectomy • Chevron osteotomy
- Distal metatarsal osteotomy • Mitchell osteotomy

KEY POINTS

- It is important to bear in mind that not one procedure is sufficient to correct all bunion deformities.
- Distal metatarsal osteotomies are indicated for the mild to moderate hallux abducto valgus deformity.
- The chevron osteotomy has acquired significant popularity and been modified throughout the years to be used in the correction of larger first intermetatarsal angles as well as correct deformities in multiplanes.
- Complications do exist for distal metatarsal osteotomies like any other surgical procedure; however, many of them are avoidable with appropriate preoperative planning, proper procedure selection, and good surgical technique.

INTRODUCTION

There have been numerous procedures described over the years for the correction of hallux abducto valgus deformities. These procedures vary from simple "bumpectomies" to first metatarsal head osteotomies to more involved basilar osteotomies and even corrective arthrodesis. Secondary to early weight-bearing, the ability to tackle deformities in multiple planes, and technical ease, the distal metatarsal osteotomies have persevered as the most popular form of correction for mild to moderate deformities. One of the most debated complications of distal metatarsal osteotomies is that of avascular necrosis (AVN). Literature supports both the prevalence of avascular necrosis following the distal metatarsal osteotomy and the lack thereof. Another complication that can cause less than desirable results is first metatarsophalangeal joint (MTPJ) stiffness.

SURGICAL TREATMENT DECISION-MAKING

There have been over 300 surgical procedures described in the literature for the correction of hallux valgus deformity. It is imperative to remember that not one

University Foot and Ankle Institute, 1919 State Street, Suite 206, Santa Barbara, CA 93101, USA
E-mail address: lindsaymaechandler@gmail.com

Clin Podiatr Med Surg 31 (2014) 221–231
http://dx.doi.org/10.1016/j.cpm.2013.12.004   **podiatric.theclinics.com**
0891-8422/14/$ – see front matter © 2014 Elsevier Inc. All rights reserved.

procedure is sufficient to correct all bunion deformities. The decision-making process must commence with the understanding that not all hallux valgus deformities are equal. When evaluating a deformity, there are many factors that must be considered. These factors include the patient's chief complaint, occupation, age, expectations, and athletic interests. Thorough physical examination of the patient's lower extremity and radiograph evaluation consisting of weight-bearing foot films are also essential in the decision-making process.

The theory that reduction of an abnormal first intermetatarsal (IM) angle is essential to hallux valgus repair is well established. A variety of bony procedures are used for correction of metatarsus primus varus. These osteotomies are located at the distal portion of the metatarsal (head and neck), the midshaft and the base of the metatarsal, and corrective arthrodesis of the first metatarsocuneiform joint. Many algorithms have been developed to provide physicians with a logical scheme with which to approach a patient with a hallux valgus deformity.

Distal metatarsal osteotomies are indicated for mild to moderate hallux valgus deformities. These procedures are intended for structural correction of the deformities of hallux abducto valgus manifested at the level of the first metatarsal head, such as increased IM angle, frontal plane rotation of the first metatarsal head, sagittal plant deformity of the first metatarsal head, and increased proximal articular set angle (PASA). Radiographically the hallux valgus angle (HVA) is less than 40°, the IM angle is less than 20°, and a there is subluxation of the first MTPJ (**Fig. 1**).

Because of several advantages, including relative ease of performance, metaphyseal location, and mechanically stable geometry, the chevron osteotomy has gained significant popularity.[1] The combination of these features facilitates rapid osseous union and early weight-bearing. Midshaft and basilar osteotomies are characteristically

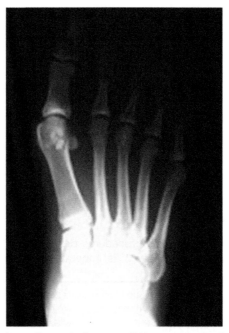

Fig. 1. An anteroposterior radiograph shows a mild increase in the first IM angle and hallux abductus angle.

indicated because the IM angle exceeds 15 to 20°. Commonly these osteotomies are accompanied by diminished intrinsic stability despite fixation, thus requiring periods of non-weight-bearing and immobilization.

HISTORICAL REVIEW
Reverdin

Reverdin[2] was the first to describe correction of hallux valgus deformity by means of a distal first metatarsal osteotomy in 1881. This procedure required a medially based wedge osteotomy in the frontal plane preserving the lateral cortex. The osteotomy is located proximal to the articular surface of the metatarsal head and distal to the sesamoid apparatus. The original intention was correction of an abnormal proximal articular set angle (PASA). This osteotomy was linked with difficult fixation and potential sesamoid disturbance.

Green[3] then described a modification to the Reverdin procedure in 1977, changing the osteotomy design to a horizontal L to evade possible damage to the dorsal articular surface of the sesamoids or the sesamoidal grooves beneath the metatarsal head. In this modification, the lateral hinge remained intact and therefore did not attend to the IM angle or sagittal plane deformities.

In 1988, Laird and coworkers[4] published another modification to the Reverdin using Green's modification as well as completing the vertical osteotomy cut by passing through the lateral cortex of the first metatarsal head and resecting a medially based wedge of bone from the plantar shaft of the metatarsal. By transposing the distal part of the first metatarsal head laterally, this modification affords a relative reduction of the metatarsus primus adductus angle as well as reducing the proximal articular set angle (PASA). The medially based wedge of bone resected would also reduce any valgus rotation of the great toe.

A year later, Zyzda and Hineser[5] used a bone graft to alleviate possible shortening as well as to correct sagittal plane deformity. They advised rotating the resected dorsal wedge of bone 180° and reinserting it into the dorsal osteotomy site with the base adjusted laterally as an autogenous bone graft to compensate for a sizable proximal articular set angle (PASA) or short first metatarsal. Likewise, the resected wedge was inserted into the plantar osteotomy with the base of the wedge lateral to account for a valgus deformity or the graft could be inserted to plantarflex the metatarsal head. These authors thought this technique avoided excessive correction and therefore overcorrection.

Today, the Reverdin is often added as an adjunct procedure to basilar osteotomies or arthrodesis to primarily account for a large PASA, most likely caused by the osteotomy's innate lack of fixation options. Lombardi and colleagues[6] described adding the Reverdin to a Lapidus procedure if soft tissue correction of the valgus deformity is deficient or the PASA is exceptionally large. However, with this combined approach considerable shortening of the first metatarsal occurs, yet Lombardi found no occurrence of lesser metatarsalgia complaints, which he attributed to sufficient plantarflexion of the metatarsal at the arthrodesis site.

Hohmann

The first surgeon accredited with describing a procedure that concurrently tackled abnormalities involving the metatarsus primus adductus angle, metatarsus primus elevatus, and the proximal articular set angle (PASA) was Hohmann. His operative technique used a complete trapezoidal osteotomy located at the anatomic neck of the first metatarsal with the widest part located medially. The location at the metatarsal neck avoided the sesamoid apparatus, decreasing the prospect of developing sesamoid arthritis. Hohmann did not believe in transecting the medial eminence; therefore, the whole procedure was performed extracapsularly. This procedure is referenced purely for a historical reference. It is no longer performed as originally depicted secondary to its unstable osteotomy and high frequency for dislocation.

Many modifications to the Hohmann procedure were fashioned to bestow more stability to the osteotomy site as well as resect the medial eminence while still attempting the same end result. In 1984, Warrick and Edelman[7] examined certain modifications such as resection of the medial eminence and altering the direction of the wedge resection to an oblique orientation rather than transverse, which permitted proper screw fixation. This modified Hohmann bunionectomy was performed on 15 feet in 11 patients. The average preoperative first IM angle was 12.5° with a postoperative angle of 7.7°. The width of the first metatarsal shaft was a limiting factor as well as the shortening that subsequently occurred when increasing the obliquity of the osteotomy to correct a greater IM angle. The amount of PASA correction was established by the size of the trapezoidal wedge resection. The authors uncovered, on average, a 4.1-mm shortening of the first metatarsal that they thought to be the most disadvantageous complication to this modified Hohmann procedure. Thus, the application of this procedure has been limited to mild to moderate hallux valgus deformities.

Mitchell

In 1945, Hawkins and colleagues[8] described a transpositional, step-cut osteotomy to correct the IM angle combined with resection of the medial eminence. It was Mitchell who later described and popularized a biplanar metaphyseal osteotomy, which displaced the capital fragment both laterally and plantarly, also shortening the first metatarsal. Merkel and colleagues[9] performed a retrospective study of 96 Mitchell first metatarsal osteotomies with an average follow-up of 7 years. Only 59% of those patients were available for follow-up. They found excessive first metatarsal shortening, dorsiflexion of the osteotomy, and failure to correct the first IM angle to 10° or less were all associated with overall patient dissatisfaction. Shortening of the first metatarsal was found to be more than 5 mm in 39 of the 56 patients available for follow-up.

The removal of a rectangular wedge of bone while attempting to retain a lateral cortical spike produces a technically demanding procedure. Significant shortening results from wedge removal that subsequently may generate lesser metatarsalgia. The threat of enhanced angulation and displacement are also probably secondary to the inherent instability of the osteotomy. Therefore, patients undergoing this procedure must be non-weight-bearing for a period of time even though most patients are able to bear weight right away following most distal metatarsal osteotomies.

Wilson

In 1963, Wilson described a through-and-through osteotomy oriented 45° from the transverse plane. This osteotomy began medially at the proximal aspect of the medial eminence and coursed in a distal-medial to proximal-lateral direction attending to the IM angle and PASA. Several complications proceeded this procedure, including shortening, inherent instability, dorsiflexion, lesser metatarsalgia, and recurrence to name a few.

Many modifications to the Wilson osteotomy ensued. Helal and colleagues[10] described orienting the osteotomy 45° to the sagittal plane, preventing dorsiflexion as well as plantarflexion of the capital fragment to compensate for any shortening. Grace and colleagues[11] reinforced the medial capsule by suturing a medial flap of capsule under tension to the periosteum or through a drill hole in the metatarsal shaft. Allen and colleagues[12] were the first to use internal fixation by placing a screw, which permitted simultaneous correction of an increased IM angle and a laterally deviated cartilaginous surface.

DRATO

Johnson and Smith[13] first described the DRATO procedure, a derotational, angulation, transpositional osteotomy of the first metatarsal head. The preoperative criteria include frontal plane rotational of the metatarsal head, abnormal proximal articular set angle (PASA), plantarward adaptation of the articular surface of the first metatarsal, mild increase of the IM angle, and a normal distal articular set angle. Because the preoperative criteria for this procedure are so specific, very few cases tend to be performed.

Chevron

In 1962, Austin first performed a horizontally directed "V" displacement osteotomy for the correction of hallux valgus. However it was not until 1981 that Austin and Leventen[1] published their description of a distal chevron osteotomy of the first metatarsal. In this publication, they reviewed more than 1200 patients in which the chevron osteotomy was performed. Their objective was to construct a procedure that addressed 3 key points: restoring the alignment of the first MTPJ, correcting the hallux valgus, and correcting the metatarsus primus varus while maintaining osteotomy stability and allowing early ambulation.

Originally this osteotomy did not include fixation. Austin thought the shape of the osteotomy as well as the impaction of the cancellous capital fragment on the shaft of the first metatarsal offered ample stability to sacrifice fixation. In 1985, Jahss and colleagues[14] assessed the operative effectiveness of 5 distinct metatarsal osteotomies for hallux valgus correction. The series had 120 feet evaluated via radiography over a 5-year period and the osteotomies included biplanar neck, chevron, biplanar basilar, basilar concentric, and basilar concentric with a lateral closing wedge. All the osteotomies with the exception of the chevron had varying plantar displacement of the capital fragment and fixation with crossed K-wires. They found the chevron gave the least amount of correction by approximately 2° and there was a 12.5% loss of correction secondary to the absence of fixation. Hattrup and Johnson[15] interviewed 154 patients with 225 chevron osteotomies: 79.1% of the procedures conveyed complete satisfaction, 12.9% stated satisfaction with minor reservations, and 8% were dissatisfied. Failure to achieve correction and technical errors were the major factors generating incomplete satisfaction.

Several modifications in the technical part of the procedure have been made since the initial depiction. These modifications have included the use of various alternative methods of internal fixation, altering the angle of the osteotomy, and augmenting with additional procedures. Numerous modifications have been created as surgeons try to benefit from the advantages of these procedures while addressing their deficiencies.

Kalish

Possibly the most popular modification to the Austin osteotomy is that of the Kalish[16] or long dorsal arm, which is more amendable to screw fixation. This modification was fashioned to address the limitations of the standard Austin procedure, including displacement and malposition of the capital fragment, delayed or nonunion, difficulties with fixation, and limited postoperative first MTPJ range of motion. The dorsal long arm osteotomy allowed for correction of larger deformities by permitting greater lateral displacement of the capital fragment. Also, 2-screw fixation was feasible, which has been found to distribute the compression forces across the osteotomy more evenly and resists rotation of the capital fragment.

Youngswick

In 1982, Youngswick[17] described a modification to the chevron osteotomy that would also plantarflex the metatarsal head for a reduction of metatarsus primus elevatus while maintaining the 60° horizontal "V" osteotomy. This modification was achieved by placing a second osteotomy parallel to the original dorsal osteotomy from the classic chevron osteotomy. This second osteotomy therefore permitted a preset portion of bone to be removed so that after impaction of the capital fragment on the metatarsal shaft, plantarflexion of the metatarsal head ensued. A true biplanar correction results when combining this modification with the lateral displacement of the classic chevron osteotomy.

Percutaneous Technique

Bösch and colleagues[18] first described a percutaneous transverse distal metatarsal osteotomy in 2000 and Giannini and colleagues[19] in 2003 and Magnan and colleagues[20] in 2005 further popularized the technique. Current trends for surgical treatment are toward minimally invasive procedures that entail minimal soft tissue stripping, theoretically decreasing morbidity. The percutaneous procedure described by Giannini and colleagues[19] begins with a 1-cm medial incision at the first metatarsal neck directly down to bone. A complete osteotomy is performed at the metatarsal neck by using an oscillating bone saw. The capital fragment is displaced to correct the hallux valgus angle (HVA), intermetatarsal angle (IMA), and distal metatarsal articular angle (DMAA) and is stabilized with a 2-mm K-wire. Their results showed no avascular necrosis of the first metatarsal head nor pseudoarthrosis of the osteotomy. The mean preoperative HVA was 33; mean preoperative IMA was 13, and the mean preoperative DMAA was 20. At an average follow-up of 7 years, the HVA was 16; IMA was 7, and the DMAA was 8.

As the distal first metatarsal osteotomies have evolved, so too have the fixation options. They comprise impaction (which in theory is not a fixation method), sutures, Kirschner wires, metallic screws, staples, absorbable screws, nonlocking plates, and locking plates. Metallic screws tend to be the most fashionable method of fixation of a distal metatarsal osteotomy. Screw fixation provides relative stability as well as compression, when inserted via a lag technique. Rotational stability may also be achieved if 2 screws are placed across the osteotomy.

OPERATIVE TECHNIQUE

Anesthesia is usually obtained with local anesthesia and intravenous sedation. An ankle pneumatic tourniquet is applied and inflated to 250 mm Hg to achieve the desired hemostasis. The incision is placed medially near the junction of the plantar and dorsal skin. This technique tends to produce a nicer cosmetic result than that of a dorsal or dorsal-medial incision. The incision is deepened by blunt dissection, taking care to retract neurovascular structures and cauterize superficial veins. A plane is created between the capsule of the first MTPJ and the subcutaneous tissue, which allows retraction of the subcutaneous tissue and its neurovascular elements as one unit. The capsulotomy is then performed using a semi-elliptical incision at the dorsomedial shoulder of the first metatarsal head and subsequently the redundant capsule is removed.

The medial eminence is resected parallel with the medial border of the foot by using an oscillating saw. The specific osteotomy is chosen and carried out in the metaphyseal region to provide a larger surface area for bone contact. The authors prefer a long dorsal arm chevron osteotomy, allowing for a 2-screw fixation, which has been found to be quite stable and decreases rotational forces (**Fig. 2**).

The metaphyseal bone aids in rapid healing and is relatively stable for fixation. In 1997, Badway and colleagues[21] reported that capital fragment following a chevron osteotomy could be displaced laterally up to 6 mm in male and 5 mm in female patients, which represents approximately 30% displacement of the metatarsal's width. However, some have advocated translating the capital fragment greater than 30% to expand the indications for the chevron osteotomy to include first IM angles in excess of 20°. In a retrospective study by Stienstra and colleagues,[22] 38 bunionectomy cases with large displacement distal chevron osteotomies (greater than or equal to 40% lateral translation) were found to have an average lateral translation of 9.8 mm with a relative change of the IM angle of 10°.

A 1.5 cm × 1.5 cm amniotic membrane graft is then placed on the dorsal aspect of the first metatarsal head and the capsule is closed with 2.0 Vicryl. Subcutaneous tissue is closed with 4.0 Monocryl and the skin is reapproximated with 5.0 nylon. Sterile compressive dressing is applied consisting of Xeroform, 4 × 4 gauze, Webril, Kling, and Coban. The tourniquet is released and the short Cam walker boot is applied while patient is still on the operating table.

POSTOPERATIVE MANAGEMENT

The patient is placed into a short Cam walker boot and is instructed to be weight-bearing as tolerated in the boot at all times. The patient's first postoperative appointment in the office is 5 days after surgery. The Cam walker boot is removed at this time and radiographs are taken in the office, including 3 views weight-bearing of

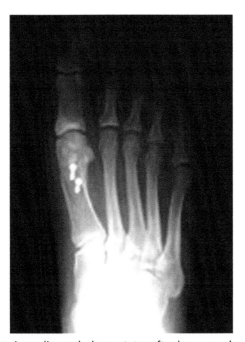

Fig. 2. An anteroposterior radiograph shows status after long arm chevron osteotomy with double-screw fixation.

the surgical foot. The bandage is changed and a fresh bandage is applied as well as the Cam walker boot. The patient is instructed to continue to weight-bear as tolerated in the boot. At 2 weeks after surgery, skin sutures are removed, allowing the patient to get incision site wet now and begin passive range-of-motion exercises about the first MTPJ. The patient continues in the short Cam walker boot for an additional 2 weeks. Radiographs are obtained again at 4 weeks after surgery, and if osseous healing is satisfactory, the patient is transitioned into a stiff-soled shoe and physical therapy may be initiated to increase the first MTPJ range of motion. Approximately 6 weeks after surgery, the patient may begin to increase activity as tolerated.

COMPLICATIONS

Just as any other surgical procedure, first metatarsal head osteotomies also have their share of possible complications. These complications can range from chronic edema to avascular necrosis of the first metatarsal head. The more common complications include delayed union, limited first MTPJ motion, lack of toe purchase, chronic edema, hallux varus/adductus, and hallux abductus. Less common complications, such as intraoperative fracture, excessive shortening, elevatus of the first metatarsal head, and avascular necrosis, may have decreased in prevalence secondary to better preoperative criteria and improved surgical instrumentation.

A common complaint after distal metatarsal osteotomies intended to treat hallux valgus is decreased first MTPJ range of motion. Jones and colleagues[23] found limited joint motion in approximately 8% of patients following head osteotomies in their retrospective statistical analysis of complications after hallux abducto valgus surgery. The authors thought the limited range of motion was secondary to first metatarsal elevates and to intracapsular adhesion.

Transfer metatarsalgia may occur secondary to excessive shortening of the first metatarsal, which in turn increases the pressure borne by the second metatarsal. Jahss and colleagues[24] state that second metatarsalgia, commonly present in conjunction with a hallux abducto valgus deformity, is further provoked by surgical procedures that shorten the first metatarsal, dorsally tilt the capital fragment, or cause loss of hallux purchase. Shapiro and Heller noted 33% of patients reported lesser metatarsalgia following a Mitchell osteotomy. Because an innate part of the Mitchell osteotomy is shortening, the authors thought the Mitchell procedure was not indicated for patients whose first metatarsal was more than 4 or 5 m shorter than the second preoperatively.[25] Conversely, Merkel and colleagues[9] found in their series of 96 Mitchell osteotomies that the primary cause of transfer metatarsalgia was dorsal displacement of the capital fragment. It is vital that the capital fragment is plantarflexed to prevent this complication.

It is essential to consider both the functional and the structural deformities of hallux valgus. When the deformity is treated surgically as only a functional or structural deformity, troubles will occur in overcorrection and undercorrection. Undercorrection or recurrence of hallux valgus is often secondary to insufficient soft tissue release or poor structural correction. The metatarsus adductus angle and the first metatarsal width are key factors when preoperatively evaluating the parameters, which will aid in the selection of the proper procedure.

It has been recorded in the literature that recurrence of hallux valgus deformity occurs in approximately 10% of cases. It is thought that this recurrence rate could be significantly lessened if the indications for the procedure are not overextended. Hattrup and Johnson[15] reported recurrence of the deformity in 18 of 225 procedures, whereby the average preoperative hallux abductus angle of 37° was corrected to an average of 31° postoperatively. Hirvensalo and colleagues[26] noted in 78 chevron osteotomies that were performed in 60 patients with painful hallux valgus, and a recurrence of the deformity occurred in 8 feet (10%). They found that hallux valgus recurred when the preoperative hallux abductus angle averaged 37° or more and the first IM angle averaged 13° or more. The risks of recurrence, undercorrection, and/or malunion are increased when using distal metatarsal osteotomies for more severe deformities.

Possibly the most severe complication is AVN. The incidence of AVN has been reported as low as 0% and as high as 20% following a distal chevron osteotomy. Jones and colleagues[27] explored the blood supply to the first metatarsal head in a cadaveric study. Using latex injection and a modified Spalteholz technique, they discovered an extraosseous network of vasculature proximal and distal to the chevron osteotomy. When the osteotomy is performed properly, both networks were preserved. Potential technical errors, such as overpenetrating the saw blade and erroneous placement of the proximal arms of the osteotomy inside the joint capsule, could cause severing of the dorsal metatarsal artery.

THE USE OF AN AMNIOTIC MEMBRANE TO AUGMENT DISTAL METATARSAL OSTEOTOMIES IN HALLUX ABDUCTO VALGUS SURGERY

The amniotic membrane is a new allograft that is procured from electively donated placentas after childbirth. This placental tissue bears unique biologic properties that promote regenerative healing while controlling inflammation and preventing scar. This bioactive matrix encloses exclusive matrix proteins that regulate inflammation and prevent scar formation, which could further lead to limited functional recovery, poor cosmesis, and further surgery.

One potentially devastating complication after first metatarsal head osteotomies is first metatarsophalangeal joint stiffness. Recently, the authors have been applying a human amniotic membrane graft to the dorsal aspect of the first metatarsal head before closure of the first metatarsophalangeal joint capsule. The authors have found this to help reduce inflammation and adhesions associated with the surgery. Patients who receive the membrane on the dorsal first metatarsal head after distal metatarsal osteotomies generally have less pain and swelling, and a better range of first MPJ motion after surgery in comparison to control patients (**Fig. 3**).

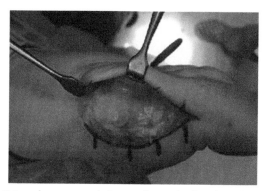

Fig. 3. A 1.5 cm × 1.5 cm human amniotic membrane is placed on the dorsal aspect of the first metatarsal head and tucked into the joint, preventing scarring and adhesions of the capsule.

SUMMARY

An array of distal first metatarsal osteotomies has been described over the decades for the correction of hallux valgus. Many of these osteotomies have been discarded or modified throughout the years. No one procedure is proficient in correcting all forms and severities of hallux valgus deformities. To optimize results, it is imperative for the surgeon to match a procedure and its modifications to the patient's deformity. The authors consider the dorsal long arm chevron osteotomy stands at the forefront for correction of mild to moderate hallux abductovalgus. The results with this specific osteotomy are predictable; it allows for early ambulation, and it is easily modified to compensate for the deformity at hand.

REFERENCES

1. Austin DW, Leventen EO. A new osteotomy for hallux valgus: a horizontally directed "V" displacement osteotomy of the metatarsal head for hallux valgus and primus varus. Clin Orthop 1981;157:25–30.
2. Reverdin J. De la deviation en dehors du gros orl (hallux valgus) et son traitement chirurgical. Trans Int Med Congr 1881;2:408–12.
3. Jenkin WM, Todd WF. Osteotomies of the first metatarsal head: reverdin, reverdin modifications, Hohmann, Hohmann modifications. In: Gerbert J, editor. Textbook of bunion surgery. 2nd edition. Mt Kisco (NY): Futura; 1991.
4. Laird PO, Silvers SH, Somdahl J. Two reverdin-laird osteotomy modifications for correction of hallux abducto valgus. J Am Podiatr Med Assoc 1988;78:403.
5. Zyzda MJ, Hinesar W. Distal L osteotomy in treatment of hallux abducto valgus. J Foot Surg 1989;28:445.
6. Lombardi CM, Silhanek AD, Connolly FG, et al. First metatarsocuneiform arthrodesis and Reverdin-Laird osteotomy for treatment of hallux valgus: an intermediate-term retrospective outcomes study. J Foot Ankle Surg 2003;42:77–85.
7. Warrick JP, Edelman R. The Hohmann bunionectomy utilizing A-O screw fixation: a preliminary report. J Foot Surg 1984;23:268–74.
8. Hawkins FB, Mitchell CL, Hedrick DW. Correction of hallux valgus by metatarsal osteotomy. J Bone Joint Surg Am 1945;27:387.
9. Merkel KD, Katoh Y, Johnson EW. Mitchell osteotomy for hallux valgus: long-term follow-up and gait analysis. Foot Ankle 1983;3:189–96.
10. Helal B, Gupta SK, Gojosen P. Surgery for adolescent hallux valgus. Acta Orthop Scand 1974;45:271.
11. Grace D, Hughes J, Klenerman L. A comparison of Wilson and Hohmann osteotomies in the treatment of hallux valgus. J Bone Joint Surg Br 1988;70:236–41.
12. Allen TR, Gross M, Miller J, et al. The assessment of adolescent hallux valgus before and after first metatarsal osteotomy. Int Orthop 1981;5:111.
13. Johnson JB, Smith SD. Preliminary report on derotational, angulational, transpositional osteotomy: a new approach to hallux abducto valgus surgery. J Am Podiatry Assoc 1974;64:667–75.
14. Jahss MH, Troy AI, Kummer F. Roentgenographic and mathematical analysis of first metatarsal osteotomies for metatarsus primus varus: a comparative study. Foot Ankle 1985;5:280–321.
15. Hattrup SJ, Johnson KA. Chevron osteotomy: analysis of factors in patients' dissatisfaction. Foot Ankle 1985;5:327–32.
16. Kalish SR. Modifications of the Austin hallux valgus repair (Kalish osteotomy). In: McGlamry ED, editor. Reconstructive surgery of the foot and leg-update '89. Tucker (GA): Podiatry Institute; 1989. p. 14–9.

17. Youngswick FD. Modifications of the Austin bunionectomy for treatment of metatarsus primus elevatus associated with hallux limitus. J Foot Surg 1982;21(2):114.
18. Bösch P, Wanke S, Legenstein R. Hallux valgus correction by the method of Bösch: a new technique with a seven- to ten-year follow-up. Foot Ankle Clin 2000;5:485–98.
19. Giannini S, Ceccarelli F, Bevoni R, et al. Hallux valgus surgery: the minimally invasive bunion correction (SERI). Tech Foot Ankle Surg 2003;2:11–20.
20. Magnan B, Pezzè L, Rossi N, et al. Percutaneous distal metatarsal osteotomy for correction of hallux valgus. J Bone Joint Surg 2005;87:1191–9.
21. Badway TM, Dutkowsky JP, Graves SC, et al. An anatomical basis for the degree of displacement of the distal chevron osteotomy in the treatment of hallux valgus. Foot Ankle 1997;18(4):213–5.
22. Stienstra JJ, Lee JA, Nakadate DT. Large displacement distal chevron osteotomy for the correction of hallux valgus deformity. Foot Ankle 2002;41:213–20.
23. Jones RO, Harkless LB, Baer MS, et al. Retrospective statistical analysis of factors influencing the formation of long-term complications following hallux abducto valgus surgery. J Foot Surg 1991;30:344–9.
24. Jahss MH. Disorders of the hallux and the first ray, ch 39. In: Jahss MH, editor. Disorders of the foot and ankle: medical and surgical management. 2nd edition. Philadelphia: WB Saunders Co; 1991. p. 943–1173.
25. Shapiro F, Heller L. The Mitchell distal metatarsal osteotomy in the treatment of hallux valgus. Clin Orthop 1975;107:225–31.
26. Hirvensalo E, Bostman O, Tormala P. Chevron osteotomy fixed with absorbable polyglycolide pins. Foot Ankle 1991;11:212–8.
27. Jones KJ, Feiwell LA, Freedman EL. The effect of chevron osteotomy with lateral capsular release on the blood supply to the first metatarsal head. J Bone Joint Surg Am 1995;77:197–204.

Scarf Osteotomy for Correction of Hallux Abducto Valgus Deformity

Lowell Weil Jr, DPM, MBA, Michael Bowen, DPM*

KEYWORDS

- Hallux abducto valgus • Hallux valgus • Bunionectomy • Metatarsal osteotomy
- Metatarsus primus varus • Scarf bunionectomy

KEY POINTS

- The scarf bunionectomy is a tricut osteotomy that can be used to correct a wide variety of intermetatarsal angles (12°–23°), abnormal proximal articular set angle values (up to 10°), and plantar or dorsal displaced metatarsals, making it a utilitarian procedure.
- The inherent stability of the scarf bunionectomy allows concurrent bilateral correction, immediate postoperative weight bearing in a surgical shoe without crutches, return to athletic shoes, and the beginning of physical therapy at 1 week after surgery.
- The long-term success, reproducibility, and ability to correct all degrees of deformity of the scarf bunionectomy have been well documented.
- Literature has shown that there is restoration of normal forefoot mechanics with the use of the scarf procedure.

INTRODUCTION

Surgical correction of hallux abducto valgus (HAV) deformity continues to be an area of interest in the foot and ankle surgical literature. Foot and ankle surgeons are continually searching for procedures that correct the multiplane deformity that occurs with HAV. With close to 130 surgical procedures described to correct the deformity, each procedure has limitations.[1] The goal of any hallux valgus surgery should be:

Long-term predictability with reproducible outcomes
To maintain a joint that is pain free with full range of motion
The ability to perform concurrent bilateral correction
Limited interference with daily activities in both the acute and long-term postoperative periods
Cosmetically pleasing result, with no restrictions in shoe gear
To provide a wide range of indications (pediatric, adult, mild to severe deformity)

Department of Podiatry, Weil Foot & Ankle Institute, 1455 Golf Road, Des Plaines, IL 60016, USA
* Corresponding author.
E-mail address: mfbowen@weil4feet.com

Clin Podiatr Med Surg 31 (2014) 233–246
http://dx.doi.org/10.1016/j.cpm.2013.12.005   **podiatric.theclinics.com**
0891-8422/14/$ – see front matter © 2014 Elsevier Inc. All rights reserved.

The scarf bunionectomy has been shown to accomplish these goals in long-term follow-up studies.[2]

The term scarf or scarf joint is used in carpentry when 2 pieces of wood are joined together and secured with the long ends overlapping. Because of its stability, the construct resists tension and compression forces (**Fig. 1**).

The Z-cut osteotomy was first introduced into bunion surgery in 1976 by Burutaran,[3] who used this procedure as an adjunct to the Keller arthroplasty for correction of hallux valgus deformity. A midshaft Z osteotomy of the first metatarsal was later revised by Gudas and Zygmunt in 1982 and then modified by Weil in 1984.[4] Borrelli and Weil[5] popularized the procedure in the United States, whereas Barouk (who learned the procedure from Weil in 1990) popularized this procedure in France, Europe, and across the world.[6] Since that time, the scarf bunionectomy has been a powerful osteotomy of the first metatarsal for the correction of HAV deformity.

Although many investigators have proposed the use of a base procedure of the first ray for the correction of moderate to severe deformities,[7] the scarf or scarf/Akin procedure remains the most widely used procedure for the correction of mild to severe hallux valgus deformity worldwide.[6,8] It has been shown to correct intermetatarsal (IM) angles approaching 23°, proximal articular set angles (PASAs) up to 10°, as well as a hallux interphalangeus angles as high as 35° when including the commonly performed adjunctive Akin procedure.[6] Indications for the scarf bunionectomy are as follows:

- Hallux valgus with a 1 to 2 IM angle of 12° to 23° (short scarf, 13° or less; medium scarf, 14°–16°; and long arm scarf, 17°–23°)
- PASA or distal metatarsal articular angle (DMAA) up to 10°
- First metatarsophalangeal joint with minimal arthritic changes, with range of motion being at least 40°

Another relative indication is that, because of the inherent stability, the scarf bunionectomy is able to be performed bilaterally in a patient requiring HAV correction without a change in the postoperative course (**Fig. 2**).

Fridman and colleagues[9] in 2009 compared the outcomes of bilateral versus unilateral correction for first ray deformities. Patients in the bilateral group returned to work faster than unilateral cases: 17.8 days versus 20.3 days, respectively. In addition, return to activities of daily living occurred sooner in the bilateral group compared with the unilateral group (15.2 vs 19.25 days, respectively), with neither providing statistical significance. The bilateral group did not have a larger complication rate and 97% of the patients having bilateral correction said they would choose that route again.

SURGICAL TECHNIQUE
Incision and Soft Tissue Release

The procedure is typically performed under monitored anesthesia care (MAC) anesthesia with a block of 20 to 25 mL of 0.5% Marcaine plain. The senior author's

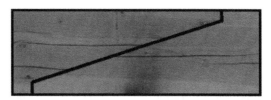

Fig. 1. Scarf joint as used in carpentry.

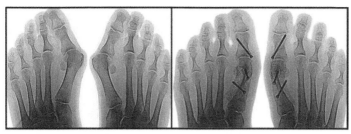

Fig. 2. Scarf bunionectomy performed simultaneously for correction of bilateral HAV deformity shown here at 6 months after surgery.

institution has found that this provides excellent postoperative analgesia, thus reducing the amount of postoperative narcotics required. This finding is anecdotal, based on experience with more than 10,000 procedures. An ankle tourniquet at 250 mm Hg is used to aid with hemostasis. The incisional approach is medial at the junction of the plantar and dorsal skin extending 5 to 7 cm from the base of the proximal phalanx to the mid to proximal first metatarsal shaft (**Fig. 3**A). The advantages of performing a medial incision approach are:

- Avoidance of the neurovascular bundles. Anatomically, the neurovascular bundle is positioned dorsal medial, which can be compromised if a dorsal medial incision is used (see **Fig. 3**B).[10] The medial incision avoids all critical neurovascular structures.
- A cosmetically pleasing scar that is not noticeable from a dorsal view (see **Fig. 3**C).
- Excellent visualization along the length of the metatarsal without putting tension on the soft tissue structures.
- The medial incisional approach, as well as the scarf cuts, minimizes disruption of the blood supply to the first metatarsal with a low incidence of osteonecrosis (**Fig. 4**A–C).

After the skin incision is deepened through subcutaneous tissue, the dorsal medial neurovascular bundle is identified and reflected. The use of urologic skin hooks allows less traumatic handling of the dorsal and plantar skin (**Fig. 5**A) and provides excellent retraction and exposure. A lenticular capsular incision is then performed, excising an

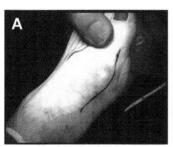
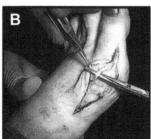
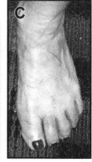

Fig. 3. (*A*) Medial incision placement along the first metatarsal. (*B*) Identification of dorsal medial neurovascular bundle. (*C*) Postoperative scar not visible from the dorsal view.

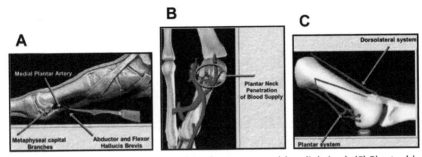

Fig. 4. (*A*) The anatomic blood supply of the first metatarsal (medial view), (*B*) Plantar blood supply, (*C*) Scarf osteotomy avoiding the anatomic blood supply. (*From* Barouk LS. Scarf osteotomy for hallux valgus correction. Local anatomy, surgical technique, and combination with other forefoot procedures. Foot Ankle Clin 2000;5:525–58; with permission.)

appropriately sized ellipse at the metatarsal head (see **Fig. 5**B). The capsule is then sharply freed, dorsally and plantarly for full visualization of the metatarsal. The skin hooks are then deepened, to reflect the capsule and skin dorsally and plantarly (see **Fig. 5**C).

An intra-articular sesamoid release is then used through the same incision with the use of a McGlammary elevator (**Fig. 6**A, B) releasing the lateral suspensory ligament. Through this approach, the blood supply to the first metatarsal is not compromised and an ancillary incision in the first interspace is not required. This technique allows for mobilization of the sesamoids and preservation of the lateral metatarsophalangeal joint ligament, thereby maintaining stability of the joint. Varus force is then placed on the hallux to ensure adequate release. Because of the power of the scarf, further lateral soft tissue release is not necessary, thereby maintaining lateral stability of the first metatarsophalangeal joint. Furthermore, the incidence of postoperative varus deformity is minimized.

Scarf Cuts

The cuts are made using an osteotomy guide, which allows consistent, reproducible, and reliable outcomes. Hetherington and colleagues[11] in 2008 found significantly different osteotomy cuts for the Austin-type cut, regardless of surgical level, when an osteotomy guide was not used. This finding has been documented in total knee arthroplasty as well as high tibial osteotomy cuts.[12,13] The scarf cuts can be oriented to produce plantar displacement, shortening, elongation, rotation, and/or translation (discussed later).

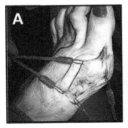
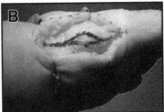
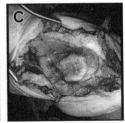

Fig. 5. (*A*) Use of urologic skin hooks for retraction. (*B*) Medial lenticular incision. (*C*) Open exposure of first metatarsal.

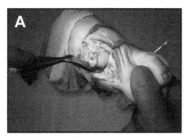
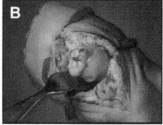

Fig. 6. (A) Insertion of McGlammary elevator plantar to first metatarsal head. (B) Releasing of lateral suspensory ligament.

Longitudinal Cut

A 1.14-mm (0.045-inch) smooth wire is inserted on the medial aspect of the first metatarsal head at approximately the dorsal one-third of the metatarsal head just proximal to the articular cartilage in the metaphyseal bone (**Fig. 7**A). The wire is directed laterally and can be angulated to create lengthening, maintain length, or create shortening as well as plantar or dorsal displacement as desired. An osteotomy guide is then inserted over the guide pin. The next step is crucial and must be performed diligently. The angle of the guide is directed toward the plantar one-third of the proximal aspect of the first metatarsal (see **Fig. 7**B).

If the proximal extent of the longitudinal cut is made too dorsal in the metatarsal, a resulting stress fracture and/or complete fracture may ensue because this is the most highly stressed area when the patient begins to bear weight.

The transverse longitudinal cut is made with a specially designed 20-mm-wide sagittal saw and osteotomy guide. Depending on the amount of lateral translation that is desired, the length of the longitudinal cut can be varied to create a short scarf

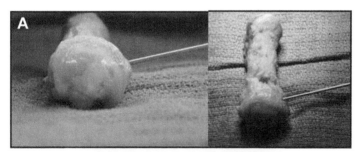

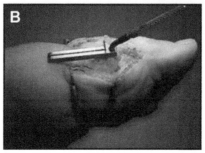

Fig. 7. (A) Angulation of smooth wire used as axis guide (shown here in a cadaver model). (B) Insertion of osteotomy guide for precise osteotomy cuts.

with IM of 13° or less; medium scarf, IM of 14° to 16°; or long-arm scarf, IM of 17° to 23°.[6] However, the senior author routinely favors the medium length scarf, even for small deformities, to ease placement of fixation.

Distal and Proximal Cut

The guide is then rotated dorsal distal around the guide pin on the metatarsal head and an angle of approximately 70° to 90° to the longitudinal cut is created in the metatarsal head. The dorsal exit point of this osteotomy is approximately 5 mm proximal to the articular surface of the first metatarsal head. It is essential to keep this distal cut in the metaphyseal bone of the metatarsal head in order to avoid troughing and channeling during the lateral displacement.[6,14] Many foot and ankle surgeons who are new to the scarf osteotomy place the cuts in the wrong location in the metatarsal, resulting in a Z osteotomy (an important difference between the scarf and the Z osteotomies is that the distal cut of the scarf osteotomy is within the metaphyseal bone of the first metatarsal head, whereas the Z places the cut in the more proximal, cortical aspect of the diametaphyseal flair of the first metatarsal **Fig. 8**). The osteotomy guide and pin are then removed from the distal apex and the horizontal and longitudinal cuts are carefully connected using the side of the saw blade.

Next, the 12-mm-wide sagittal saw blade is used to make the proximal cut (**Fig. 9**), which is typically oriented at 45° to 60° to the longitudinal cut. This cut should be oriented in the same direction as the distal alignment pin.

Once the osteotomy has been completed, a push-pull technique is used to create correction. The plantar shelf is then translated laterally and the dorsal shelf pulled medially by the use of a phalangeal clamp (**Fig. 10**A). Once appropriate correction is obtained, a scarf clamp (see **Fig. 10**B) is introduced plantarly (a phalangeal clamp can also be used), rotated dorsally, and secured in place for temporary fixation.

Fixation

Distal fixation is obtained using a 2.5-mm, partially threaded, headless compression screw. The distal screw is inserted distal to the scarf clamp and aimed plantarly and distally toward the crista in the head of the first metatarsal with care not to penetrate the plantar cortex of the metatarsal head. The proximal screw is also a 2.5-mm, partially threaded, headless compression screw. This screw is inserted proximal to the scarf clamp, dorsal medial on the first metatarsal, and aimed lateral plantar to capture the plantar shelf for bicortical fixation (**Fig. 11**). The scarf clamp is then removed.

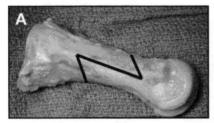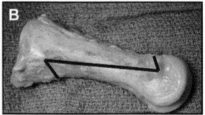

Fig. 8. (*A*) Z osteotomy, with equal amounts of dorsal and plantar bone in the diaphysis. (*B*) Scarf osteotomy, which shows a more distally based cancellous cut in the metaphysis, the distal cut in the dorsal one-third of the metatarsal and the proximal cut in the plantar one-third of the metatarsal, and the overall increase in length of the diaphyseal cut (the diaphyseal cut should be made parallel to the weight-bearing surface).

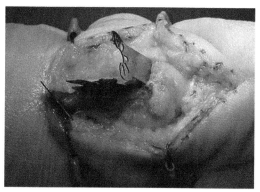

Fig. 9. Scarf osteotomy cuts with appropriate angles both proximally and distally in relation to the horizontal cut.

Adjunctive Procedure: Akin Osteotomy

The hallux is then examined to determine whether an Akin osteotomy is needed. With the hallux placed in line with the first metatarsal, creating a congruent joint, the interphalangeal deformity is assessed. If an interphalangeal deformity is present, an Akin procedure is performed. It has been noted that the Akin osteotomy is performed in close to 90% of the scarf bunionectomies performed by the senior author, which is similar to other studies.[1,15,16] The Akin osteotomy aligns both the flexor hallucis longus (FHL) and extensor hallucis longus (EHL) tendons, which not only aligns the vector of the tendons' pull within the first ray but also produces a more cosmetically pleasing outcome. The procedure is a closing base wedge osteotomy on the medial aspect of the proximal phalanx of the hallux. The phalanx is approached through an extension of the same medial incision used during the scarf procedure.

DeMore and colleagues[17] in 2012 found the average insertion of the flexor hallucis brevis (FHB) onto the proximal phalanx base to be 7 mm. The Akin osteotomy is performed 8 to 10 mm distal to the articular surface of the proximal phalanx, thereby

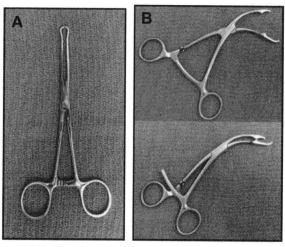

Fig. 10. (*A*) Phalangeal clamp, (*B*) open and closed scarf clamp.

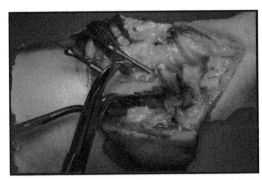

Fig. 11. Scarf clamp used for temporary fixation, and insertion of two 2.5-mm screws in appropriate orientation as described earlier. Note the significant lateral translation of the capital fragment.

avoiding the insertion and not compromising the function of the FHB. Protection of the FHL and EHL tendons is paramount, and this can be done by placement of a Freer elevator (or similar retractor) dorsally and plantarly between the phalanx and the tendons. In addition, the distal interphalangeal joint can be plantarflexed during the osteotomy to allow for laxity of the FHL. The proximal cut is made parallel to the base of the proximal phalanx keeping the lateral cortex intact. The distal cut is then made and an appropriately size triangular wedge of bone is removed. The osteotomy is then fixated with one 2.5-mm partially threaded screw as shown in **Fig. 12**.

In addition, the redundant bone on the medial portion of the first metatarsal head and shaft is removed with a sagittal saw in line with any bony overhang while the joint is held in a rectus position. A rotary burr is then used to remodel and smooth the dorsomedial aspect of the metatarsal head and the medial metatarsal shaft. The incision is then thoroughly irrigated.

Closure

A capsuloplasty is accomplished with a 2-0 absorbable suture, placing the suture immediately medial to the tibial sesamoid and connecting it to the dorsal portion of the capsule using a pulley suture technique (**Fig. 13**). This suture configuration is 2.5 times stronger than a simple suture. The toe is held in a rectus position during capsular closure, ensuring that there is no residual deformity or overcorrection. The capsuloplasty is critical to realign the first metatarsal sesamoid articulation.

This factor has been postulated to be important in prevention of recurrent bunion deformities.[18] Skin is then closed with a subcuticular 5-0 absorbable suture (**Fig. 14**A). The incision is then reinforced with 12.7-mm (0.5-inch) Steri-Strips. A bulky compressive bandage is then applied with the hallux and first ray in its corrected position (see **Fig. 14**B). A 15-cm (6 inch) compressive bandage is applied with sequential compression from the metatarsal heads to midcalf and a surgical shoe is dispensed.

ADJUNCTS AND MODIFICATIONS
Plantar Displacement

If 15° of plantar displacement is desired, the smooth wire should aim to the plantar aspect of the fifth metatarsal. If 20° of plantar displacement is desired, the K-wire should be aimed toward the plantar aspect of the fourth metatarsal (**Fig. 15**).

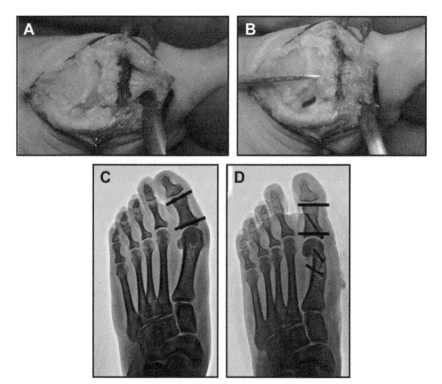

Fig. 12. (A) Removal of triangular-shaped wedge from proximal phalanx. (B) Closure of the Akin (lateral cortex still intact). (C) Preoperative Akin (note the incongruous lines). (D) Postoperative Akin (note that the lines are more parallel).

Lengthening/Shortening

Shortening is obtained by directing the smooth guidewire from distal medial to proximal lateral on the first metatarsal. The osteotomy guide follows that direction and, as the capital fragment is moved laterally, it slides down the slope and creates shortening of the first metatarsal segment. If significant shortening is needed, a small wedge of

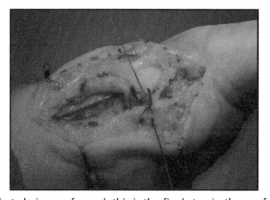

Fig. 13. Capsuloplasty being performed; this is the final step in the scarf bunionectomy.

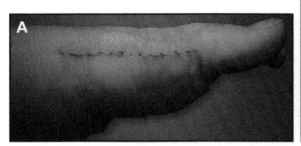
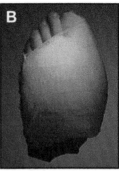

Fig. 14. (A) Subcuticular closure with absorbable suture provides a cosmetically appealing scar, and eliminates the need for removal of sutures at the postoperative visit. (B) Compressive bandage applied for postoperative edema control; note that the bandage is applied with the first ray in its relaxed position without overcorrection.

bone is removed from both the dorsal distal cut as well from the plantar proximal cut. In the unlikely event that lengthening is needed, the smooth guidewire is directed proximal medial to distal lateral and the capital fragment moves up the slope in this circumstance.

Correction PASA

Up to 10° of rotation can be obtained for correction of PASA (DMAA). This correction is accomplished by excising a medially based triangular wedge of bone from the dorsal cut with the apex being directed laterally (**Fig. 16**). The proximal portion of the metatarsal swings more laterally within the first interspace and both IM correction and transverse rotation can be accomplished with this variation.

Postoperative Course

Time period: 0 to 7 days

Patients are discharged from the facility once stable with a surgical shoe on each foot that underwent a procedure. Immediate guarded weight bearing without the use of crutches or a cane is allowed whether unilateral or bilateral procedures were performed. Patients are advised to limit activities during the first week and should only

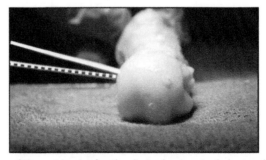

Fig. 15. Angulation of the guidewire for the desired amount of plantar displacement of the capital fragment. The dotted line is directed toward the fifth metatarsal, and the solid line is directed toward the fourth metatarsal for more plantar displacement.

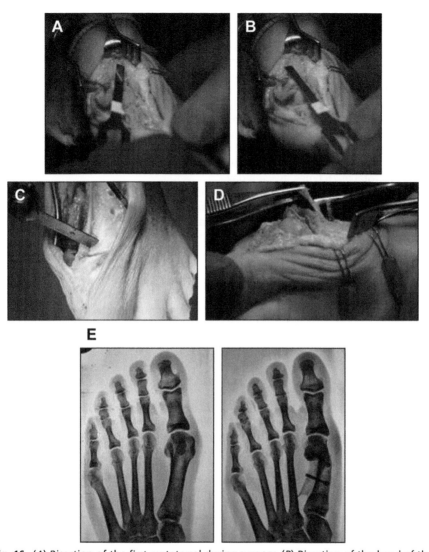

Fig. 16. (*A*) Bisection of the first metatarsal during surgery. (*B*) Bisection of the head of the first metatarsal during surgery (note the disparity of angles between *A* and *B*). (*C*) Angulation of dorsal cut to correct PASA (DMAA) (note that the apex is lateral on the metatarsal). (*D*) Removal of wedge. (*E*) Decrease in PASA (DMAA) after removal of bone wedge.

be on their feet to use the washroom and to get something to eat. Patients are prescribed nonsteroidal antiinflammatory drugs for 7 days after surgery. This antiinflammatory regimen is augmented with moderate analgesic drugs if necessary. Patients are instructed to remove the compressive bandage daily, but to avoid disturbing the dressings beneath. While the compressive bandage is off, patients are to perform range-of-motion exercises of both the subtalar and ankle joint to minimize musculature and joint contractures, followed by 10 minutes of icing and then reapplication of the compressive bandage.

Time period: 7 days to 6 weeks

Patients return for the first postoperative visit at 7 to 10 days after surgery. At that time all bandages are removed and they are placed back into their own running/athletic shoes. At this visit, formal physical therapy is instituted with an aggressive home program. This program includes using passive stretching of the first metatarsophalangeal and strengthening of all movements, but particular attention is directed to flexion strength of the FHL tendon. The use of an elastic band around the great toe with the ankle held at 90° provides the best mechanical advantage of strengthening of the FHL and FHB tendons against resistance. Patients are dispensed a brace that reduces swelling and also has elastic attachments to help develop strength of the great toe (**Fig. 17**). Patients should perform the flexion exercises for 3 sets of 25 each for a total of 75 times, twice a day.

Malinoski and colleagues[19] presented a poster at the American College of Foot and Ankle Surgery Annual Scientific Conference in Las Vegas in 2010, and Schuh and colleagues[20] in 2010 investigated formal physical therapy following bunion surgery. Both groups found significant improvement in both pain and function in patients receiving formal physical therapy programs.

Patients are allowed to bathe immediately, but are instructed not to soak the surgical foot. They are also instructed that the only time they can come out of the athletic sneakers are for bathing, sleeping, and doing their physical therapy program because the sneakers provide a barrier against excessive swelling. Patients are also allowed to drive a car as soon as they feel comfortable to do so.

Time period: 6 weeks to 3 months

If radiographic and clinical healing are progressing, patients are allowed to transition into a greater variety of shoe gear, including dress shoes and high heels. Patients can also begin low-impact activities (eg, walking, treadmill, and elliptical machine) but can progressively increase their activities based on overall comfort, and some can return to more high-impact activities. There is continued emphasis on home physical therapy programs for strengthening and stretching. The patients are instructed to continue with antiinflammatory medication if there is any residual pain or swelling.

Time period: 3 months to 1 year

Patients return to regular activities and there are no restrictions in shoe gear. Antiinflammatories are ceased, but strengthening and stretching are still encouraged daily depending on the patient's strength and range of motion. Minimal swelling should be noted at this point.

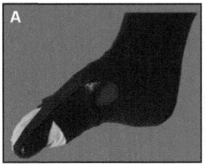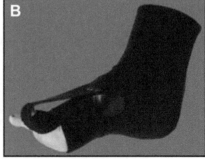

Fig. 17. Edema-controlling braces with flexion straps that provide resistance at maximal plantar-flexion (*A*) and maximal dorsi-flexion (*B*). As strength increases, the straps can be anchored further back on the foot, providing more resistance.

Complications

The scarf bunionectomy is a technically challenging procedure with a steep learning curve.[8,21] As with all surgical procedures, the scarf bunionectomy has the risk of surgical complications but the senior author has developed techniques to minimize these.

The most commonly cited complication of the scarf bunionectomy has been stated to be troughing. Coetzee[21] reported a 35% complication of troughing in 2003, but the procedure shown in that study is more in line with the Z osteotomy than the scarf bunionectomy. His follow-up study in 2007 reported only 2 cases in 187 feet, which is a significantly lower rate than in his initial work.[22] This lower rate is more consistent with the lack of troughing reported in a case series of 3567 feet published in 2000 by Weil.[6]

Other reported complications include the following:

- Six percent recurence[23]
- Between 3% and 5% hallux varus[4,6,24]
- Five percent removal of painful fixation[6]
- Three percent stress fractures, which significantly decreased after 1995[6]
- Two percent loss of correction[6]
- Two percent metatarsalgia[6]

PATIENT SATISFACTION

Overall, the scarf bunionectomy has yielded high patient satisfaction rates after surgery. Weil[6] found that 92% of the patients would have the surgery again, 5% with some reservation, and only 3% would not have the procedure again.

Patient-reported outcomes have yielded excellent results, and have provided significant improvements in postoperative mean AOFAS (American Orthopaedic Foot and Ankle Society) scores, ranging from 86 to 96.1.[1,23–26] Also, significant reductions (6°–10°) in IM 1 to 2 angles as well as reduction of the hallux valgus angle (15°–26°)[1,6,15,24–26] have been shown.

SUMMARY

The scarf osteotomy has been used and researched extensively for many years for the correction of hallux valgus deformity in both the adolescent and adult populations. It is an inherently stable construct, which allows for early weight bearing and early return to activities of daily living. The scarf procedure has a wide array of surgical indications with great reproducibility and a low complication rate, and it can be performed bilaterally simultaneously, with long-term predictability. Once the scarf procedure is mastered, it is a rewarding and predictable operation for both the surgeon and patient.

REFERENCES

1. Jones S, Al Hussainy HA, Ali F, et al. Scarf osteotomy for hallux valgus. A prospective clinical and pedobarographic study. J Bone Joint Surg Br 2004;86: 830–6.
2. Berg RP, Olsthoorn PG, Poll RG. Scarf osteotomy in hallux valgus: a review of 72 cases. Acta Orthop Belg 2007;73:219–23.
3. Burutaran JM. Hallux valgus y cortedad anatomica del primer metatarsano (correction quirurgica). Actual Med Chir Pied 1976;13:261–6.
4. Zygmunt KH, Gudas CJ, Laros GS. Z-bunionectomy with internal screw fixation. J Am Podiatr Med Assoc 1989;79:322–9.

5. Borrelli AH, Weil LS. Modified scarf bunionectomy: our experience in more than one thousand cases. J Foot Surg 1991;30:609–12.

6. Weil LS. Scarf osteotomy for correction of hallux valgus. Historical perspective, surgical technique, and results. Foot Ankle Clin 2000;5:559–80.

7. Trnka HJ, Muhlbauer M, Zembsch A, et al. Basal closing wedge osteotomy for correction of hallux valgus and metatarsus primus varus: 10- to 22-year follow-up. Foot Ankle Int 1999;20:171–7.

8. Barouk LS. Scarf osteotomy of the first metatarsal in the treatment of hallux valgus. Foot Dis 1995;2:35–48.

9. Fridman R, Cain JD, Weil LJ, et al. Unilateral versus bilateral first ray surgery: a prospective study of 186 consecutive cases–patient satisfaction, cost to society, and complications. Foot Ankle Spec 2009;2:123–9.

10. Solan MC, Lemon M, Bendall SP. The surgical anatomy of the dorsomedial cutaneous nerve of the hallux. J Bone Joint Surg Br 2001;83:250–2.

11. Hetherington VJ, Kawalec-Carroll JS, Melillo-Kroleski J, et al. Evaluation of surgical experience and the use of an osteotomy guide on the apical angle of an Austin osteotomy. Foot (Edinb) 2008;18:159–64.

12. Minns RJ. Surgical instrument design for the accurate cutting of bone for implant fixation. Clin Mater 1992;10:207–12.

13. Odenbring S, Egund N, Lindstrand A, et al. A guide instrument for high tibial osteotomy. Acta Orthop Scand 1989;60:449–51.

14. Barouk LS. Scarf osteotomy for hallux valgus correction. Local anatomy, surgical technique, and combination with other forefoot procedures. Foot Ankle Clin 2000;5:525–58.

15. Lorei TJ, Kinast C, Klarner H, et al. Pedographic, clinical, and functional outcome after scarf osteotomy. Clin Orthop Relat Res 2006;451:161–6.

16. Crevoisier X, Mouhsine E, Ortolano V, et al. The scarf osteotomy for the treatment of hallux valgus deformity: a review of 84 cases. Foot Ankle Int 2001;22:970–6.

17. Demore M, Baze E, Lalama A, et al. The anatomical location of the flexor hallucis brevis as it pertains to implant arthroplasty. J Am Podiatr Med Assoc 2012;102:1–4.

18. Okuda R, Kinoshita M, Yasuda T, et al. Postoperative incomplete reduction of the sesamoids as a risk factor for recurrence of hallux valgus. J Bone Joint Surg Am 2009;91:1637–45.

19. Malinoski KA, Weil L, Weil LS, et al. Retrospective comparison of patients undergoing formal physical therapy versus no physical therapy following bunion correction. Poster, ACFAS National meeting. Las Vegas (NV). February 22–26, 2010.

20. Schuh R, Hofstaetter SG, Adams SB, et al. Rehabilitation after hallux valgus surgery: importance of physical therapy to restore weight bearing of the first ray during the stance phase. Phys Ther 2009;89:934–45.

21. Coetzee JC. Scarf osteotomy for hallux valgus repair: the dark side. Foot Ankle Int 2003;24:29–33.

22. Coetzee JC, Rippstein P. Surgical strategies: scarf osteotomy for hallux valgus. Foot Ankle Int 2007;28:529–35.

23. Kristen KH, Berger C, Stelzig S, et al. The SCARF osteotomy for the correction of hallux valgus deformities. Foot Ankle Int 2002;23:221–9.

24. Choi JH, Zide JR, Coleman SC, et al. Prospective study of the treatment of adult primary hallux valgus with scarf osteotomy and soft tissue realignment. Foot Ankle Int 2013;34:684–90.

25. Adam SP, Choung SC, Gu Y, et al. Outcomes after scarf osteotomy for treatment of adult hallux valgus deformity. Clin Orthop Relat Res 2011;469:854–9.

26. Lipscombe S, Molloy A, Sirikonda S, et al. Scarf osteotomy for the correction of hallux valgus: midterm clinical outcome. J Foot Ankle Surg 2008;47:273–7.

First Metatarsal Base Osteotomies for Hallux Abducto Valgus Deformities

Jason Morris, DPM, AACFAS[a],*, Michael Ryan, DPM[b]

KEYWORDS

- Proximal • Bunion • Wedge • Base • Hallux valgus • Crescentic

KEY POINTS

- Proximal first metatarsal osteotomies allow effective correction of hallux abducto valgus deformities by correcting closer to the apex of deformity.
- Common complications are nonunion, first metatarsal elevation, difficulty with fixation, and first metatarsal shortening.
- Opening wedge plates and crescentic osteotomies provide significant deformity correction with minimal shortening or even lengthening of the metatarsal.
- Advances in fixation have allowed predictable results and have limited the complications commonly associated with proximal osteotomies.

Selection of the appropriate surgical procedure for hallux valgus deformities relies on many factors and the large variation of osteotomies provides surgeons with seemingly unlimited surgical options. The hallux abducto valgus deformity incorporates many entities that must be acknowledged when surgical intervention is considered. Increase in intermetatarsal angle, hallux abductus angle, mobility of the first ray, patient age, patient health status, activity level, previous surgical procedures, surgeon skill level, and so forth are all factors in determining the best procedural choice. The goal is to restore functional, physiologic anatomy and to minimize complications, providing the patient with a long-lasting successful outcome.

A protocol for hallux valgus surgery that used to be commonly used is distal osteotomy for intermetatarsal angles of less than 13° to 15° and proximal osteotomy for angles greater than 13° to 15°. However, selecting the appropriate procedure is more complicated than radiographic evaluation and intermetatarsal angle. This process is as complex as the cause and characteristics of the deformity. As understanding of the hallux valgus deformity has continued to progress, procedural options have also

[a] University Foot and Ankle Institute, 2121 Wilshire Boulevard Suite 101, Santa Monica, CA 90403, USA; [b] Private Practice, 2021 Freeport Road, Arnold, PA 15068, USA
* Corresponding author.
E-mail address: drjmorris@footankleinstitute.com

Clin Podiatr Med Surg 31 (2014) 247–263
http://dx.doi.org/10.1016/j.cpm.2013.12.006
0891-8422/14/$ – see front matter © 2014 Elsevier Inc. All rights reserved.
podiatric.theclinics.com

advanced. Adaptations of osteotomies, improvements in surgical technique, and use of procedure-specific hardware have made proximal first metatarsal osteotomy an appealing procedure for correction of hallux valgus deformities. For this reason, proximal metatarsal osteotomies should not necessarily be limited to the traditional procedural selection criteria of large intermetatarsal angles.

INDICATIONS
Large Intermetatarsal Angles

The most common application of a proximal metatarsal procedure for hallux valgus correction is with a large intermetatarsal angle. In the past, this was considered for measurements greater than 13° to 15°. Distal osteotomies tend to have an inherent limitation of translation because they are restricted by the width of the metatarsal shaft. In general, it is recommended that distal osteotomies should not exceed 25% to 50% translation in relation to the metatarsal shaft. Exceeding this translation leads to instability of the capital fragment and limitations on fixation.[1,2] Jahss and colleagues[3] evaluated the geometric principles of first metatarsal osteotomies. With a distal chevron type osteotomy, instability of the construct occurred with any intermetatarsal angle correction greater than 5°. In comparison, a proximal osteotomy allowed greater correction because the center of rotation is closer to the origin of deformity.[4]

Because the correction occurs proximally and closer to the axis of rotation, a greater level of correction can be obtained using proximal procedures.[5] The geometric placement of the osteotomy allows for a greater distance between the hinge and the most distal point of the metatarsal. A longer radius arm creates a greater lateral correction of the distal metatarsal for each degree of correction at the proximal osteotomy site, which allows the first metatarsal head to come in closer proximity to the second metatarsal and thus reduces the intermetatarsal angle to a greater extent.

Jahss[6] discussed general geometric principles in relation to metatarsal osteotomies. In translational or transpositional osteotomies such as a chevron, for each 1 mm of lateral displacement of the distal portion of the osteotomy there is 1 mm of intermetatarsal angle. Both distal and proximal translational osteotomies result in the same amount of correction of metatarsus primus varus. Because of this, they recommended limiting this type of osteotomy to intermetatarsal angles of less than 12°. For rotational osteotomies, such as the crescentic procedure, a base osteotomy has 5 times greater transverse plane effect on the metatarsal head compared with a neck osteotomy. Jahss[6] showed that 15° of rotation at the metatarsal neck results in 2.5° of correction, but 12.5° of correction when performed at the metatarsal base. Wedge osteotomies provide a closer ratio of correction. A 5-mm closing or opening wedge at the neck and base provide approximately 7.5° and 10.25° of correction, respectively. The amount of correction, especially in base procedures, also depends on the length of the first metatarsal because a longer lever arm allows a greater amount of intermetatarsal reduction when performed close to the axis of correction.[6]

Short First Metatarsal

Although shortening of the metatarsal is a common result of some base osteotomies, such as the closing base wedge, other procedures allow minimal shortening or lengthening of the metatarsal. The crescentic osteotomy has traditionally been an osteotomy that provided minimal shortening. Because the osteotomy relies on closure of the intermetatarsal angle through rotation along the osteotomy as opposed to removal of bone, shortening is limited to the thickness of the osteotomy blade plus any amount of blade excursion. In a retrospective review of 75 patients, Mann and colleagues[7] saw an average of 2 mm of shortening at a mean follow-up of 34 months.

Opening wedge osteotomies also have the ability of deformity correction without shortening of the first metatarsal. However, in the past, this type of osteotomy was bypassed in favor of closing base wedge osteotomies for large metatarsus primus varus deformities because of the limitation in internal fixation. With the improvement of fixation options and the advent of opening wedge plates, the proximal first metatarsal opening wedge osteotomy has gained popularity over the last several years. Opening wedge plates not only allow the surgeon to avoid shortening the metatarsal but also make lengthening possible (**Fig. 1**). Bundy and colleagues[8] showed that approximately 1% to 3% of lengthening can be expected with opening wedge base osteotomies. Other studies have shown average lengthening between 2.3 mm and 2.6 mm with the use of opening wedge plates.[9,10] Although a concern of metatarsal lengthening is transfer pain, both of these studies confirmed the absence of transfer metatarsalgia after opening wedge osteotomy.

Hypermobile First Ray

Excessive hypermobility of the first metatarsocuneiform joint has not only been shown to be a causative component of hallux valgus but also affects the structural mechanics of the foot.[11,12] An insufficient first ray can be linked to excessive pronation, overload of the lesser metatarsals, and abnormal motion of the first metatarsophalangeal joint. Signs of hypermobility include a flexible forefoot varus, diffuse hyperkeratosis under the second or third metatarsal heads, metatarsalgia, recurrent

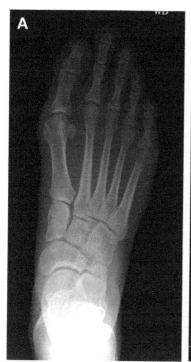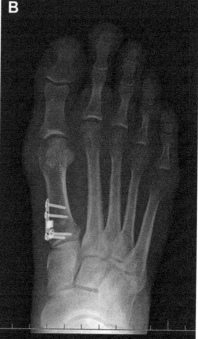

Fig. 1. (*A*) Indication for opening wedge plate, short first metatarsal. (*B*) Correction of deformity with opening wedge plate.

lesser metatarsal stress fractures, thickening of the second metatarsal shaft, and subluxation of the second metatarsophalangeal joint.[13]

Gellman and colleagues[14] showed normal sagittal plane range of motion of the first metatarsocuneiform joint to be 5.7° of dorsiflexion and 5.8° of plantarflexion. Lee and colleagues[15] determined normal total range of motion of the first ray to be 10.3° and it was measured at 12.9° in patients with hallux valgus. Although hypermobility was a previously identified entity of foot biomechanics, it was Lapidus[16] who first described hypermobility of the first tarsometatarsal joint and a correlation to hallux valgus. Because of this connection he recommended fusion of the joint as a way to address the excessive mobility. Fusion of the joint has endured as the procedure of choice for hypermobility of this joint.

More recent research provides a different insight into the relationship between excessive mobility of the first ray and hallux valgus deformity. Rush and colleagues[17] showed a reduction in first ray mobility with the use of a proximal metatarsal osteotomy and concluded that first ray stability was linked to realignment of the windless mechanism. This finding showed that first ray hypermobility may not be simply a characteristic of the first metatarsocuneiform joint, but more a function of first ray alignment. Coughlin and colleagues[18] and Coughlin and Jones[19] were able to show a decrease in first ray hypermobility, but with use of a proximal crescentic osteotomy and distal soft tissue realignment. The study showed approximately 50% decrease in sagittal plane mobility of the metatarsocuneiform joint, from 11 mm to 5.2 mm. It is this malalignment and subsequent loss in windlass effect that may have a greater impact on mobility of the first ray than the first tarsometatarsal joint.

CLOSING BASE WEDGE OSTEOTOMY
Overview

The first described osteotomy at the base of the first metatarsal was by Loisin in 1901. In 1903, Balacescu was the first to perform a proximal osteotomy, but it was not until later in the twentieth century that closing base wedge osteotomies gained popularity. This popularity coincided with improvements in internal fixation. By 1981, Youngswick[20] described the closing base wedge osteotomy as the most popular procedure for severe hallux abducto valgus. The osteotomy was traditionally created in a transverse orientation, using fixation with Kirschner wires (**Fig. 2**).

The Juvara modification of the closing base wedge, which uses an obliquely oriented osteotomy, was implemented to increase contact surface and points of fixation. In recent years, the popularity of the closing base wedge osteotomy has diminished in part because of concerns of shortening. A 10-year to 22-year follow-up study showed an average shortening of 5 mm.[21] Concerns also exist about stability of the osteotomy. If the medial hinge is left intact, the cortical bone provides additional stability. However, if the hinge is lost, the osteotomy becomes intrinsically unstable and deforming forces are not transferred across the osteotomy, which occurs in a chevron-type osteotomy.[22]

Technique

The first metatarsophalangeal joint is approached through a standard dorsal incision. The medial eminence is exposed and removed with an oscillating saw. The lateral soft tissues are released, including the capsule, lateral sesamoid ligament, and adductor hallucis brevis tendon. Extending the incision or making a separate incision to the first metatarsocuneiform joint allows access to the proximal osteotomy site (**Fig. 3**). The incision length can vary depending on the choice of fixation.

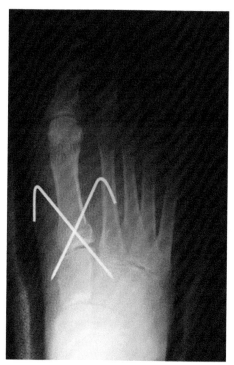

Fig. 2. Closing base wedge osteotomy. Osteotomy is transverse, which poses an inherent difficulty with fixation.

Using a 1.14-mm (0.045-inch) guide K-wire, the medial hinge is marked 1 to 1.5 cm distal to the metatarsocuneiform joint and the appropriate-sized wedge is removed using saw resection. If an oblique osteotomy is created, the hinge is placed approximately 5 mm from the medial edge of the first metatarsal base and directed at a 45° to 65° angle to the long axis of the first metatarsal. Using an oscillating or sagittal saw the distal bone cut is made followed by the proximal bone cut perpendicular to the weight-bearing surface with care to maintain the medial hinge. Do not attempt closing the osteotomy until after the guidewire is removed to reduce the risk of fracturing the medial cortex. A reciprocating motion can be used with the bone saw along the medial hinge to allow gradual closure of the osteotomy and good bone apposition.

If sagittal plane correction is required to compensate for excessive shortening, the medial hinge can be transected and the distal fragment rotated plantarly. Distal translation of the osteotomy can also be performed to lengthen the first metatarsal after closure of the wedge osteotomy. Keep in mind that by sacrificing the medial hinge, the stability of the osteotomy can be compromised. Without appropriate fixation, unwanted postoperative rotation or translation may occur.

Under fluoroscopic guidance, the osteotomy is stabilized with internal fixation. Different fixation techniques using K-wires, Steinman pins, screws, and plates have been described. Fillinger and colleagues[23] showed 2-screw fixation to be more stable than single-screw fixation. Using standard Arbeitsgemeinshaft fur Osteosynthesefragen (AO) technique, compression screws or a low-profile locking plate can be used to address torsion, bending, and tension across the osteotomy (**Fig. 4**).[22] Once fixated, a distal osteotomy may be required to correct proximal articular set angle.

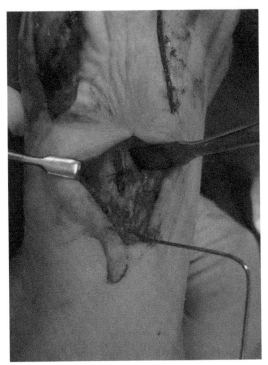

Fig. 3. Access to the proximal first metatarsal base through a separate proximal incision. Medial distal incision created for access to the first metatarsophalangeal joint.

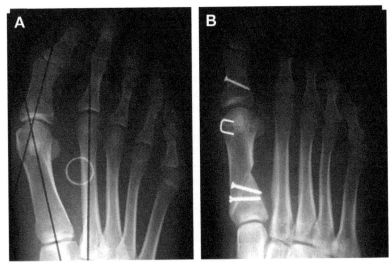

Fig. 4. (*A*) Preoperative hallux abducto valgus deformity. (*B*) Postoperative deformity correction with oblique proximal closing wedge osteotomy, Akin osteotomy, and distal wedge correction of proximal articular set angle.

OPENING WEDGE OSTEOTOMY
Overview

The opening base wedge technique was first described by Trethowan[24] in 1923, in which stability was maintained with intact lateral hinge and wedge graft. Because of concern with first metatarsophalangeal joint jamming from lengthening, Stamm[25] recommended a concomitant Keller arthroplasty to eliminate this concern. He used the bone from the proximal phalanx base for use as bone graft in the opening wedge. Beronio[26] described using the medial eminence of the first metatarsal head as a graft for the opening wedge osteotomy.

This osteotomy is powerful in reducing the intermetatarsal angle and can also increase metatarsal length. In the retrospective study of 47 patients, the average intermetatarsal angle was reduced from 16° to 8° after surgery.[27] Shurnas and colleagues[28] found 3.2° of intermetatarsal angle correction per millimeter of wedge and 1.8 mm of metatarsal length gain. As mentioned previously, approximately 2 to 3 mm of first metatarsal lengthening can be expected depending on the size of wedge used. This lengthening can result in tightening of the soft tissues surrounding the first metatarsophalangeal joint and predispose it to jamming and decreased range of motion.[28,29]

A historical disadvantage of the opening base wedge osteotomies has been the requirement of internal fixation, which was suboptimal. As technology has advanced from a simple unthreaded wire to fixed-angle constructs, this concern has lessened and popularity has increased. Attention has now shifted to early weight bearing with the use of opening wedge plates, specifically locking plate designs (**Table 1**). In Smith and colleagues'[27] review of 47 patients the average time to begin partial weight bearing was 13.5 days, and they recommended a locked plate system if attempting an aggressive postoperative weight bearing protocol. Wukich and colleagues[10] started heel weight bearing at 2 weeks and progressed to full weight bearing as tolerated with a boot and crutches at 4 weeks with no transfer lesions reported in 18 cases. Saragas and colleagues[9] started their patients on heel weight bearing in a wedged shoe with crutches/walker for the first 2 weeks in 64 cases, of which 1 developed a nonunion.

Technique

Using a dorsal or medial incision, the first metatarsal head is accessed and the medial eminence is resected. The lateral soft tissues are released accordingly. A separate

Table 1			
The most commonly used opening wedge plates			
	Screw Design	Screw Size (mm)	Wedge Size (Interval)
Synthes/Depuy	Locking (variable angle)	2.4, 2.7	0, 3–7 mm (1 mm)
Wright (Darco)	Locking, nonlocking	2.7, 3.5	0–7 mm (1 mm)
Arthrex	Locking, nonlocking	2.4	2–7 mm (0.5 mm)
Paragon 28	Locking, nonlocking	2.7	0, 3–8 mm (1 mm)
Vilex	Locking	2.5	3–6 mm (1 mm)
Osteomed	Locking (variable angle), nonlocking	2.7	0, 2–5 mm (0.5 mm)
Stryker	Locking, nonlocking	3.0, 3.5	0, 3–5 mm (1 mm)
Merete	Locking	3.0, 3.5	0, 2–6 mm (2 mm)
Orthohelix	Locking, nonlocking	2.7, 3.5, 4.0	2–6 mm (1 mm)

incision or extended incision can be used to create the proximal osteotomy. The author's preferred technique is through a separate medial incision, which allows access to the osteotomy site and placement of an opening wedge plate along the medial first metatarsal base.

The osteotomy is created 1 to 1.5 cm distal to the metatarsocuneiform joint into metaphyseal bone with an oscillating or sagittal saw. The cut is made from medial to lateral with an attempt to maintain the lateral cortex. This result can be achieved with the use of a guidewire to mark the hinge. The generally recommended technique is to perform the osteotomy halfway between perpendicular to the metatarsal and the weight-bearing surface. Hardy and colleagues[29] recommended making this cut perpendicular to the weight-bearing surface, because they think this results in less sagittal plane elevation. An osteotome can be used to carefully open the wedge, with care to keep the lateral hinge intact (**Fig. 5**). If using an opening wedge plate for fixation, most systems include an instrument to facilitate opening of the osteotomy. Fluoroscopy should be used to observe correction of the intermetatarsal angle and reduction of the sesamoid position.[27]

Described fixation techniques include K-wires and staples but the most common fixation has been low-profile wedge plates (**Fig. 6**). The increase in popularity is secondary to the increased stability, use of variable wedge sizes, and ability for early weight bearing.[9,10,27] Wedge spacers range in size from 2 mm to 7 mm and are determined by the size of the deformity. Recommendations include inserting the distal screw close to the osteotomy to allow stabilization of the osteotomy to the plate.[9,10] The opening wedge can be filled with autograft from the medial eminence resection or allograft bone.

PROXIMAL CHEVRON OSTEOTOMY
Overview

The proximal chevron procedure is a horizontal V osteotomy of the first metatarsal base. That was first described by Kotzenberg[30] in 1929, but more popularized by Sammarco and colleagues[30] and Easley and colleagues.[31] Because of the dorsal and plantar arms of the osteotomy, the proximal chevron has some inherent stability that can be lacking in other proximal osteotomies. It is this sagittal plane stability that

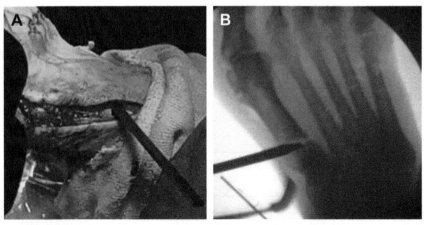

Fig. 5. (*A, B*) Use of osteotome to open medial aspect of metatarsal for opening wedge osteotomy.

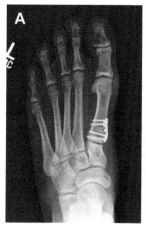
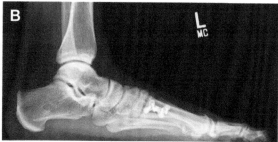

Fig. 6. (*A, B*) Anteroposterior and lateral radiographs after correction with locking, opening wedge plate.

can limit complications such as dorsiflexion. Easley and colleagues[31] performed a prospective, randomized, comparative study between proximal crescentic and proximal chevron osteotomies. This study showed a shorter healing time and less metatarsal shortening with the chevron osteotomy. Dorsiflexion malunion is a problematic complication seen in some proximal base procedures, in particular with the crescentic osteotomy. This finding was seen in 17% of the crescentic osteotomies versus 0% in chevron osteotomy.[31]

Technique

Similar to other proximal osteotomies, a distal incision is created in order to resect the medical eminence. The proximal V osteotomy is made 1 cm to 2 cm distal to the metatarsocuneiform joint. A longitudinal incision is created medial and midaxial over the base of the first metatarsal. The incision is typically 4 to 5 cm in length, but may vary in order to achieve adequate exposure and can be an extension of the distal incision. Medial dorsal and plantar sensory nerves should be protected as well as the extensor hallucis longus tendon dorsally. The apex of the osteotomy is marked 1.5 cm distal to the metatarsocuneiform joint. The arms of the osteotomy are made at 45° to 60° to each other and may be directed proximally or distally depending on the surgeon's preference. If angled proximally, the osteotomy may be created slightly distally to allow for fixation without intrusion of the metatarsocuneiform joint. If the osteotomy extends too proximally it can intrude into the capsular region of the point and make translation of the osteotomy more difficult.

Once the osteotomy is completed, the distal portion can be translated laterally and temporarily fixated in order to visualize reduction of the deformity. Translation of the osteotomy can be facilitated by providing medial force on the proximal fragment with the use of a clamp. At this point, some surgeons prefer to angle or slightly impact the osteotomy at the lateral aspect to allow further correction of the intermetatarsal angle. Because the translational osteotomy is limited by the amount of space between the bases of the first and second metatarsals, angulation can improve reduction of the deformity. Although helpful in deformity correction, this can also make the osteotomy less stable and increase difficulty in fixation. Borton and Stephens[32] described the use of a dorsal medial wedge graft for angulation of the osteotomy as opposed to increased compression along the lateral aspect of the osteotomy site. This technique also allows slight plantarflexion at the osteotomy site to adjust for potential shortening and dorsiflexion. Allograft can be used, but some surgeons have advocated the use of the resected portion of the medial eminence as the graft.[32]

Several variations of fixation have been recommended for this osteotomy. Although initially described without fixation, the use of screws allows a more stable construct than with Kirschner wires or staples alone.[33] The most common construct is 1 or 2 screws placed dorsally from distal to proximal. Sharma and colleagues[34] used a plantar-to-dorsal screw placement in a cadaveric study and showed increased stability using this screw orientation compared with a dorsal-to-plantar screw. They advocated that, with the incision location being medial, a plantar-placed screw is no more technically difficult than one placed dorsally. Supplemental transverse K-wire fixation has been described to improve stability.[35] Easley and colleagues[36] recommended the use of a medial locking plate because it provided good stability and allowed early weight bearing.

CRESCENTIC OSTEOTOMY
Overview

Popularized by Mann and colleagues[7] in the early 1990s, the proximal crescentic osteotomy uses a crescentic or arcuate bone cut. Deformity correction is achieved through rotation of the distal fragment along the osteotomy site. With a rotational osteotomy, correction of the deformity can easily be adjusted by either medial or lateral rotation of the distal fragment to make minor adjustments without the necessity of additional bone cuts or grafts while limiting shortening.

The crescentic osteotomy was originally described as a through-and-through cut of the metatarsal base. The major problem with this technique was difficulty in fixation. Because of this, instability and dorsiflexion malunion were the major pitfalls of the procedure (**Fig. 7**). In Mann and colleagues'[7] original studies they reported a malunion

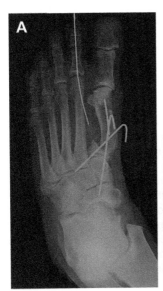
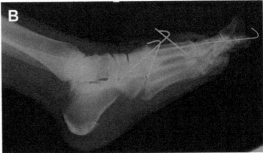

Fig. 7. (A, B) Inadequate fixation of crescentic osteotomy resulting in shifting of the osteotomy and subsequent malunion.

rate of 28%. Despite this, patients had a 93% satisfaction rate. Veri and colleagues[37] used a similar technique, resulting in 94% patient satisfaction over a 12.2-year follow-up. Thordarson and Leventen[38] reported a 93.5% satisfaction rate among 33 cases with an average follow-up of 28 months.

Variations of the crescentic osteotomy were developed to limit these complications. The most widely used modification of the osteotomy is a crescentic shelf procedure, which was originally described by Cohen and colleagues.[39] This procedure converts the crescentic osteotomy into a more stable and reproducible construct by combining a dorsal-to-plantar crescentic osteotomy and a medial-to-lateral transverse osteotomy at the base of the metatarsal. The plantar shelf is created to facilitate fixation options while maintaining the precise corrective ability of the rotational osteotomy and limiting shortening. Stability of the osteotomy site is the key component in reducing or eliminating malunion of the crescentic osteotomies. Fixation options include K-wires, screws, and dorsal plates.

Technique

The medial eminence is addressed per typical protocol. The proximal crescentic osteotomy is performed through a dorsal, longitudinal incision over the base of the first metatarsal. A 3-cm to 4-cm incision is normally required, but may be lengthened depending on fixation choice or adjunctive procedures. The osteotomy is performed 1 to 1. 5 cm distal to the tarsometatarsal joint with a crescentic blade. The crescentic blade is available in several sizes and is chosen based on the width of the metatarsal. The osteotomy can be created with the concave surface facing distally or proximally. Several investigators advocate having the convex surface face distally to dissipate the retrograde deforming forces at the osteotomy site.[40] Doing so also allows greater bone contact along the osteotomy site and eliminates the medial prominence created by the rotated base of the distal fragment.

Using the blade, the osteotomy is created from dorsal to plantar and perpendicular to the weight-bearing surface. This technique allows movement of the distal fragment laterally without unwanted dorsal or plantar movement. The blade is gradually rotated back and forth in a medial-to-lateral rotation along the inherent arch of the blade. If the blade is too narrow compared with the metatarsal, it is best to complete the osteotomy through the lateral cortex and use a straight blade to transect the medial cortex. Because the osteotomy is rotated laterally, the medial cortex does not factor into the osteotomy correction. Attempting to complete the osteotomy laterally in this situation may not only affect the correction but puts the comminuting artery between the base of the first and second metatarsals at risk.[36]

The crescentic shelf osteotomy is a variation of the procedure that provides added stability and room for fixation. The created shelf may be a long or short arm depending on the fixation desired. A long plantar shelf allows for multiple screws that aid in rotational stability in addition to sagittal plane stability. When using a plantar shelf, the surgeon should create the plantar osteotomy first in a medial-to-lateral direction in the plantar one-third of the metatarsal bone. Care should be taken to make this as close to parallel as possible to the weight-bearing surface. A K-wire can be placed to guide the osteotomy in the correct orientation. This technique is helpful because abnormal deviation of the saw blade either medially or laterally in the coronal plane can result in abnormal sagittal plane movement at the osteotomy. The crescentic blade is then used to create the osteotomy in the dorsal two-thirds of the metatarsal using the technique described earlier.

Once the osteotomy is created the distal fragment is rotated laterally (**Fig. 8**). This fragment is visualized using intraoperative fluoroscopy to avoid overcorrection. To

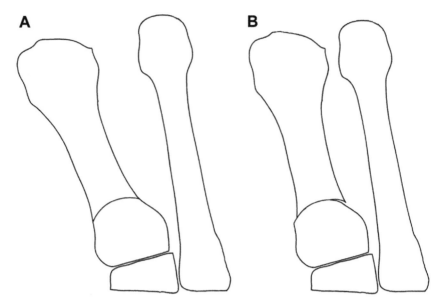

Fig. 8. (*A, B*) Crescentic osteotomy and correction of metatarsus primus varus deformity.

facilitate positioning of the osteotomy, the proximal metatarsal fragment can be pulled laterally with a bone hook or clamp. Kirchner wires are used for temporary fixation. Permanent fixation is placed consisting of wires, screws, or a plate. Many clinicians have recommended use of a dorsal plate as the primary or supplementary fixation because of its increased strength and load to failure compared with single-screw fixation.[41–43]

COMPLICATIONS

As with any procedure, complications are of big concern when choosing the appropriate surgical plan. When dealing with common disorders such as hallux abducto valgus deformities, complications are common. Whether performing a distal, mid-shaft, or proximal metatarsal procedure, similar complications are to be expected such as hallux varus, recurrence, or joint stiffness. The complications most commonly associated with proximal metatarsal osteotomies are discussed later. Delayed union, shortening, elevation, and injury to the dorsalis pedis artery are the most problematic complications specific to this procedural subset.

Nonunion/Delayed Union

Nonunions are of concern with any osteotomy, including those performed during correction of a hallux valgus deformity. Potential reasons for a nonunion in proximal osteotomies of the first metatarsal include vascular injury, thermal necrosis, infection, inadequate fixation, or excessive tension forces at the osteotomy site. Smith and colleagues[27] reported an 8% rate of delayed union or nonunion with use of a nonlocking opening wedge plate and 0% when using a locking plate design (**Fig. 9**). With closing wedge osteotomies, reported nonunion rates have been low with few to no reports of union complications.[44–46] This finding is most likely secondary to the larger bone contact area with an oblique osteotomy and multiple points of fixation. The crescentic osteotomy has reported consistently low rates of nonunion despite varying rates of malunion.[7,37,47]

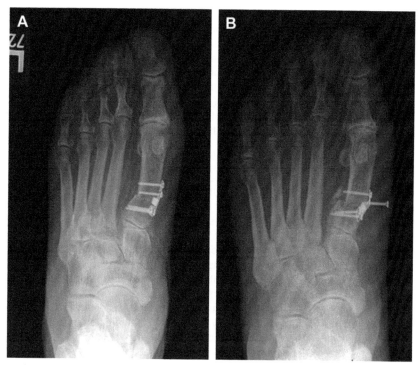

Fig. 9. (*A, B*) Fixation with nonlocking plate and hardware failure resulting in malunion and delayed union of opening wedge osteotomy site.

Vascular Injury

With any osteotomy at the proximal first metatarsal, the dorsalis pedis artery is at increased risk of injury. The dorsalis pedis artery is a continuation of the anterior tibial artery. It courses along the dorsal aspect of the midfoot and divides into the deep plantar artery and first dorsal metatarsal artery in the proximal aspect of the first metatarsal interspace. This division typically occurs 10 mm distal to the first metatarsocuneiform joint.[48] The deep plantar artery passes between the bases of the first and second metatarsal bones in a dorsal-proximal to plantar-distal direction. It forms the plantar arterial arch in combination with the lateral plantar artery.

The plantar arch provides blood supply to the metatarsal heads and toes.[49] Chuckpaiwong and Korwutthikulrangsri[50] performed an anatomic study evaluating the safe zone for proximal osteotomies of the first metatarsal head. Dorsally along the first metatarsal, the artery is present approximately 1.2 cm from the joint. Plantar, the artery is at risk 2.3 cm from the joint, which creates a triangular-shaped safe zone at the first metatarsal base, which is typically only of concern with osteotomies that break the lateral cortex of the first metatarsal, such as in the proximal chevron, closing wedge, and crescentic osteotomies.

Shortening

Shortening is a complication with many osteotomies, especially when there is wedge resection for deformity correction. Banks and colleagues[51] used mathematical and experimental models to determine metatarsal shortening with closing base wedge osteotomies. Osteotomies of 5°, 10°, and 15° resulted in shortening of 1.1 mm, 1.7 mm, and 2.5 mm, respectively. Day and colleagues[44] found a 2.2-mm average shortening in first metatarsal length with closing base wedge osteotomies. In a mathematical model, Kummer[4] showed 2.6 mm of average shortening. It is this significant change in length that makes minimal shortening osteotomies of the first metatarsal base appealing in the surgical setting. Sammarco and colleagues[30] measured approximately 2 mm of metatarsal shortening with a proximal chevron osteotomy. Computer analysis showed shortening of 1 mm with the crescentic osteotomy, although slightly more shortening should be expected with saw blade excursion and possible bone resorption.[52]

Elevation

Elevation of the first metatarsal is a result of dorsiflexion malunion of proximal first metatarsal osteotomies or poor surgical technique. The crescentic procedure has historically been associated with the highest rate of malunion. Several studies have reported malunion rates with this osteotomy. Percentages of dorsiflexion malunion have been reported at 28% for Mann and colleagues,[7] 17% for Easley and colleagues,[31] and 9% for Zettl and colleagues.[47] Thordarson and Leventen[38] found an average of 6.2° of dorsiflexion with crescentic osteotomies. Pearson and colleagues[53] saw an average of 7.1 mm of dorsal displacement. Studies have shown a direct correlation between medial-to-lateral coronal tilt with the osteotomy and elevation of the metatarsal.[54,55] Modifications of this osteotomy, changes in fixation, and increased awareness of complications have resulted in a lower rate of dorsiflexion malunion.

Even in other proximal osteotomies, elevation has been a common complication. Schuberth and colleagues[56] identified elevation of the first metatarsal in 93.7% of patients who had closing based wedge osteotomies. Despite this, they were unable to determine whether the elevation was from the intraoperative setting or postoperative migration. Wanivenhaus and Felder-Busztin[57] noted a 60% incidence of dorsal displacement with this osteotomy. With dorsal angulation at the osteotomy, transfer metatarsalgia is of great concern. Although Mann and colleagues[7] noted that dorsiflexion of the first metatarsal did not influence transfer lesions, others have reported incidences of transfer metatarsalgia at 40% or more.[21]

SUMMARY

The ideal osteotomy for a bunion deformity is one that corrects intermetatarsal angle and hallux abductus angle while avoiding unwanted complications. Proximal metatarsal osteotomies can be a good procedural choice for correction of hallux valgus deformities. In the past, these procedures have been hindered by complications and limitations such as delayed union, malunion, long periods of immobilization, and high requirement of technical skill. Improvements in fixation and technique allow successful use of proximal osteotomies and limit these complications. Osteotomies of the proximal metatarsal should be considered for a wide range of hallux valgus deformities and hold benefits that allow expanded use beyond severe deformities.

REFERENCES

1. Austin DW, Leventen EO. A new osteotomy for hallux valgus. Clin Orthop Relat Res 1981;157:25–30.
2. Corless JR. A modification of the Mitchell procedure. J Bone Joint Surg Br 1976; 58:128–32.

3. Jahss MH, Troy AI, Kummer FJ. Roentgenographic and mathematical analysis of first metatarsal osteotomies for metatarsus primus varus: a comparative study. Foot Ankle 1985;5(6):280–321.
4. Kummer FJ. Mathematical analysis of first metatarsal osteotomies. Foot Ankle 1989;9(6):281–9.
5. Ruch JA. Base wedge osteotomies of the first metatarsal. In: McGlamary ED, Banks AS, Downey MS, editors. Comprehensive textbook of foot surgery, vol. I, 2nd edition. Baltimore (MD): Williams & Wilkins; 1992. p. 504–22.
6. Jahss MH. Disorders of the hallux and the first ray. In: Jahss MH, editor. Disorders of the foot & ankle: medical and surgical managementvol. II, 2nd edition. Philadelphia: WB Saunders; 1991. p. 943–1174.
7. Mann RA, Rudicel S, Graves SC. Repair of hallux valgus with a distal soft-tissue procedure and proximal metatarsal osteotomy. A long term follow-up. J Bone Joint Surg Am 1992;74(1):124–9.
8. Bundy AM, Masadeh SB, Lyons MC II, et al. The opening base wedge osteotomy and subsequent lengthening of the first metatarsal: an in vitro study. J Foot Ankle Surg 2009;48(6):662–7.
9. Saragas NP. Proximal opening-wedge osteotomy of the first metatarsal for hallux valgus using a low profile plate. Foot Ankle Int 2009;30(10):976–80.
10. Wukich DK, Rousell AJ, Dial DM. Correction of metatarsus primus varus with an opening wedge plate: a review of 18 procedures. J Foot Ankle Surg 2009;48(4): 420–6.
11. Hirsch BE. Structural biomechanics of the foot bones. J Am Podiatr Med Assoc 1991;81(7):338–43.
12. Ito H, Shimizu A, Miyamoto T, et al. Clinical significance of increased mobility in the sagittal plane in patients with hallux valgus. Foot Ankle 1999;20(1): 29–32.
13. Myerson MS, Badekas A. Hypermobility of the first ray. Foot Ankle Clin 2000; 5(3):469–84.
14. Gellman H, Leniham M, Halikis N, et al. Selective tarsal arthrodesis: an in vitro analysis of the effect on foot motion. Foot Ankle 1987;8(3):127–33.
15. Lee KT, Young K. Measurement of first ray hypermobility in normal vs hallux valgus patients. Foot Ankle Int 2001;22(12):960–4.
16. Lapidus PW. Operative correction of the metatarsus varus primus in hallux valgus surgery. Surg Gynecol Obstet 1934;58:183–91.
17. Rush SM, Christensen JC, Johnson CM. Biomechanics of the first ray. Part II: metatarsus primus varus as a cause of hypermobility. A three-dimensional kinematic analysis in the cadaver model. J Foot Ankle 2000; 39(2):68–77.
18. Coughlin MJ, Jones CP, Viladot R, et al. Hallux valgus and first ray hypermobility: a cadaveric study. Foot Ankle Int 2004;25(8):537–44.
19. Coughlin MJ, Jones CP. Hallux valgus and first ray mobility: a prospective study. J Bone Joint Surg Am 2007;89(9):1887–98.
20. Youngswick FD. Closing abductory wedge osteotomy of the first metatarsal base. In: Gerbert J, editor. Textbook of bunion surgery. New York: Futura Publishing; 1981. p. 237–50.
21. Trnka HJ, Muhlbauer M, Zernbsch A, et al. Basal closing wedge osteotomy for correction of hallux valgus and metatarsus primus varus: 10 to 22 year follow-up. Foot Ankle Int 1999;20(3):171–7.
22. Sammarco VJ, Acevedo J. Stability and fixation techniques in first metatarsal osteotomies. Foot Ankle Clin 2001;6(3):409–32.

23. Fillinger EB, McGuire JW, Hesse DF, et al. Inherent stability of proximal first metatarsal osteotomies: a comparative analysis. J Foot Ankle Surg 1998; 37(4):292–302.
24. Trethowan J. Hallux valgus. In: Choyce CC, editor. A system of surgery. New York: PB Hoeber; 1923. p. 1046–9.
25. Stamm TT. The surgical treatment of hallux valgus. Guys Hosp Rep 1957;106(4): 273–9.
26. Beronio JP. One approach to a viable method of obtaining cancellous bone for grafting. J Foot Surg 1983;22:240–2.
27. Smith WB, Hyer CF, DeCarbo WT, et al. Opening wedge osteotomies for correction of hallux valgus: a review of wedge plate fixation. Foot Ankle Spec 2009; 2(6):277–82.
28. Shurnas PS, Watson TS, Crislip TW. Proximal first metatarsal opening wedge osteotomy with a low profile plate. Foot Ankle Int 2009;30(9):865–72.
29. Hardy MA, Grove JR. Opening wedge osteotomy of the first metatarsal using the Arthrex low profile plate and screw system. Foot Ankle Online J 2009; 2(4):2.
30. Sammarco GJ, Brainard BJ, Sammarco VJ. Bunion correction using proximal chevron osteotomy. Foot Ankle 1993;14(1):8–14.
31. Easley ME, Kiebzak GM, Davis WH, et al. Prospective, randomized comparison of proximal crescentic and proximal chevron osteotomies for correction of hallux valgus deformity. Foot Ankle Int 1996;17(6):307–16.
32. Borton DC, Stephens MM. Basal metatarsal osteotomy for hallux valgus. J Bone Joint Surg Br 1994;76(2):204–9.
33. Lian G, Markolf K, Cracchiolo A. Strength of fixation constructs for basilar osteotomies of the first metatarsal. Foot Ankle 1992;13(9):509–14.
34. Sharma KM, Parks BG, Nguyen A, et al. Plantar-to-dorsal compared to dorsal-to-plantar screw fixation for proximal chevron osteotomy: a biomechanical analysis. Foot Ankle Int 2005;26(10):854–8.
35. Amis JA, Porter DM. Correction augmentation and provisional fixation in proximal metatarsal osteotomies using Kirschner wires. Foot Ankle Int 1999;20(11): 752–3.
36. Easley ME, Darwish HH, Schreyack DW, et al. Proximal first metatarsal osteotomies. In: Saxena A, editor. International advances in foot and ankle surgery. London: Springer; 2012. p. 11–25.
37. Veri JP, Pirani SP, Claridge R. Crescentic proximal metatarsal osteotomy for moderate to severe hallux valgus: a mean 12.2 year follow-up study. Foot Ankle Int 2001;22(10):817–22.
38. Thordarson DB, Leventen EO. Hallux valgus correction with proximal metatarsal osteotomy: two year follow-up. Foot Ankle 1992;13(6):321–6.
39. Cohen M, Roman A, Ayres M, et al. The crescentic shelf osteotomy. J Foot Ankle Surg 1993;32(2):204–26.
40. Carpenter B, Motely T. Adding stability to the crescentic basilar first metatarsal osteotomy. J Am Podiatr Med Assoc 2004;94(5):502–4.
41. Rosenburg GA, Donley BG. Plate augmentation of screw fixation of proximal crescentic osteotomy of the first metatarsal. Foot Ankle Int 2003;24(7):570–1.
42. Chow FY, Lui TH, Kwok KW, et al. Plate fixation for crescentic metatarsal osteotomy in the treatment of hallux valgus: an eight year followup study. Foot Ankle Int 2008;29(1):29–33.
43. Varner KE, Matt V, Alexander JW, et al. Screw versus plate fixation of proximal first metatarsal crescentic osteotomy. Foot Ankle Int 2009;30(2):142–9.

44. Day T, Charlton TP, Thordarson DB. First metatarsal length change after basilar closing wedge osteotomy for hallux valgus. Foot Ankle Int 2011;32(5):513–8.
45. Seiberg M, Felson S, Colson JP, et al. Closing base wedge versus Austin bunionectomies for metatarsus primus adductus. J Am Podiatr Med Assoc 1994; 84(11):548–63.
46. Pontious J, Mahan KT, Carter S. Characteristics of adolescent hallux abducto valgus. A retrospective review. J Am Podiatr Med Assoc 1994;84(5):208–18.
47. Zettl R, Trnka HJ, Easley M, et al. Moderate to severe hallux valgus deformity: correction with proximal crescentic osteotomy and distal soft tissue release. Arch Orthop Trauma Surg 2000;120(7–8):397–402.
48. Lee JH, Dauber W. Anatomic study of the dorsalis pedis-first dorsal metatarsal artery. Ann Plast Surg 1997;38(1):50–5.
49. Rath B, Notermans HP, Franzen J, et al. The microvascular anatomy of the metatarsal bones: a plastination study. Surg Radiol Anat 2009;31(4):271–7.
50. Chuckpaiwong B, Korwutthikulrangsri E. Safety area for proximal metatarsal procedures. Foot Ankle Int 2013;34(4):579–81.
51. Banks AS, Cargill RS II, Carter S, et al. Shortening of the first metatarsal following closing base wedge osteotomies. J Am Podiatr Med Assoc 1997; 87(5):199–208.
52. Kay DB, Njus G, Parish W, et al. Basilar crescentic osteotomy: a three-dimensional computer simulation. Orthop Clin North Am 1989;20(4):571–82.
53. Pearson SW, Kitaoka HB, Cracchiolo A, et al. Results and complications following a proximal curved osteotomy for the hallux metatarsal. Contemp Orthop 1991;23(2):127–32.
54. Jones CP, Coughlin MJ, Viladot R, et al. Proximal crescentic metatarsal osteotomy: the effect of saw blade orientation on first ray elevation. Foot Ankle Int 2005;26(2):152–7.
55. Lippert FG, McDermott JE. Crescentic osteotomy for hallux valgus: a biomechanical study of variables affecting the final position of the first metatarsal. Foot Ankle 1991;11(4):204–7.
56. Schuberth JM, Reilly CH, Gudas CJ. The closing wedge osteotomy: a critical analysis of first metatarsal elevation. J Am Podiatr Med Assoc 1984;74(1):13–24.
57. Wanivenhaus AH, Feldner-Busztin H. Basal osteotomy of the first metatarsal for the correction of metatarsus primus varus associated with hallux valgus. Foot Ankle 1988;8(6):337–43.

Fixation Updates for Hallux Valgus Correction

Rotem Ben-Ad, DPM

KEYWORDS

- Fixation • Hallux valgus • Bunion • Kirschner wire • Staple • Screw • Plate

KEY POINTS

- Repair of hallux valgus deformities is a mainstay procedure in every surgical foot and ankle practice.
- Many different fixation devices and constructs can all yield identical surgical outcomes.
- The trend toward more stable internal fixation has allowed for earlier rehabilitation and return to function after surgery.

INTRODUCTION

Repair of hallux valgus deformities is a mainstay procedure in every surgical foot and ankle practice. Although most procedures performed for the correction of bunion deformities share a common foundation, each foot and ankle surgeon differs slightly in his or her approach to providing the patient with the most optimal surgical outcome. Procedural choices, dissection techniques, fixation methods, and postoperative regimens vary from practitioner to practitioner. In terms of fixation, an almost identical result can be achieved by using many different types of fixation techniques and devices.

As in every facet of medicine and surgery, there have been considerable advances in the nature of fixation devices available for the surgical repair of hallux valgus deformities. The internal fixation options for osteotomies and fusions are now vast considering what existed only 20 years ago. In fact, the original Austin bunionectomy was described without the use of any internal fixation.[1] However, with the growing belief in stable internal fixation as popularized by the AO Foundation, the acceptable methods of performing osteotomies and fusions have evolved throughout the years. The trend toward more stable internal fixation has allowed for earlier rehabilitation and return to function after surgery. In fact, the evolution of certain fixation structures with the use of plates has even permitted early weight bearing in patients who undergo fusions. The alternatives for internal fixation in the correction of hallux valgus are reviewed in this article.

University Foot and Ankle Institute, 2121 Wilshire Boulevard, Suite 101, Santa Monica, CA 90403, USA
E-mail address: rbenad@gmail.com

Clin Podiatr Med Surg 31 (2014) 265–279
http://dx.doi.org/10.1016/j.cpm.2013.12.008
0891-8422/14/$ – see front matter © 2014 Elsevier Inc. All rights reserved.

CERCLAGE AND KIRSCHNER WIRE FIXATION
Cerclage Wiring

The most primitive form of fixation is most probably the use of cerclage wiring. Although not the first choice for most hallux valgus procedures, cerclage and tension band techniques do still find their place in the right circumstances. Cerclage wiring entails the use of flexible wire encircled around an osteotomy or fracture site. Although not ideal, the cerclage technique does afford some level of interfragmentary compression. Probably the most useful application of cerclage wiring is in patients with severely osteoporotic bone where screw purchase is unlikely.[2] Secondly, cerclage methods may be used as a bail out technique in a scenario where the primary form of fixation has failed.

The main procedure cerclage wiring may still be used for as the principle form of fixation is the Akin osteotomy. The most stable construct for the Akin procedure is with an osteotomy that is oriented transversely.[3] Orienting one cut of the wedge parallel to the appropriate joint surface also provides the most accurate correction of the deformity. This, however, results in a transverse osteotomy once the wedge is removed. The transverse orientation is obviously not conducive to screw fixation. Cerclage wiring may therefore be a viable option. Generally, a 26- or 28-gauge monofilament wire is used. The most stable construct when using cerclage wiring to fixate an Akin osteotomy is to pass the loop through four cortices.[3] Load studies using saw bone models have shown that using a dorsal two-cortices technique results in only the dorsomedial cortex being compressed, and the osteotomy is unable to resist axial loads adequately.[4] Providing increased stability, a wire passing four cortices as a vertical loop perpendicular to the plane of the osteotomy is recommended.[3] A horizontal loop can also be used but this requires a greater amount of soft tissue dissection.[3] In both techniques, the surgeon must rely on an intact lateral cortical hinge for added stability. Although some interfragmentary compression is acquired, this method does not result in rigid internal fixation and therefore caution should be taken with weight bearing. Fixation of a metatarsal osteotomy with cerclage is also possible but is not currently considered the ideal choice by most surgeons. Nevertheless, it may prove to be a useful technique to have in one's arsenal if the primary form of fixation has failed and a bail out option is necessary (**Fig. 1**).

Transfixation with Kirschner Wires

The main benefits to using Kirshner wires (also known as K-wires) are their ease of use and low level of cost. Although they do afford some stability across an osteotomy or fusion site, they do not provide the advantage of interfragmentary compression. K-wires allow for adequate resistance to motion perpendicular to the wire. However, when the movement is parallel to the wire, they offer little use.[5] Rigidity can be significantly increased by placing two K-wires at 90° to one another.[2] Wires can be found with both smooth and threaded tips, with the threaded version providing slightly more stability. Aside from lack of rigid compression, another disadvantage of K-wire fixation is the heat generated with insertion. Some argue that this may lead to bone necrosis and is caused by the absence of real cutting facets and flutes.[2] Studies have shown that thinner wires (<1.1 mm) generate less heat than thicker ones, and that diamond-tip wires generate less heat than smooth or trocar-tip wires.[2] Regardless of these issues, K-wires have continued to be a tried and true method of fixation for many applications in hallux valgus surgery. One other option available if wire fixation is desired is absorbable pins. These can be used in the same fashion as an ordinary K-wire, but negate the need for possible removal in the future.

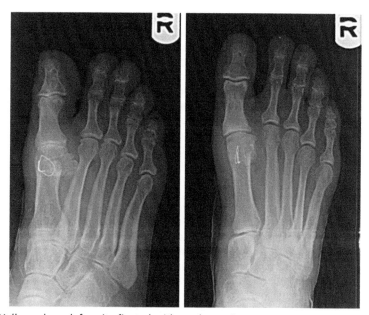

Fig. 1. Hallux valgus deformity fixated with cerclage wire.

One of the more simple procedures for use of wire fixation is again the Akin osteotomy (**Fig. 2**). If the surgeon is able to preserve the lateral cortical hinge, minimal sacrifice in fixation is made by using a single K-wire. Generally, a 0.045 or 0.062 wire is used and some advantage is gained by using a threaded K-wire. By allowing the wire to penetrate both cortices, the maximum amount of stability is achieved.[3] If the lateral hinge does unfortunately break, a second K-wire can be inserted in a crossed fashion to provide the necessary security for the osteotomy. Depending on the exact configuration and the skin incision made the K-wire may either be cut flush and buried, or left exposed to be removed at a later date. In their study, Chacon and colleagues[4]

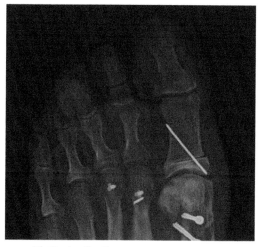

Fig. 2. Akin osteotomy with K-wire fixation.

compared the biomechanical stability of different fixation techniques of the Akin osteotomy in sawbone models. They found crossed Kirschner wires as having the greatest load to failure and deemed this construct the most mechanically stable.

Fortunately, many of the metatarsal osteotomies for hallux valgus repair performed today are inherently stable and therefore conducive to fixation solely with K-wires. Probably the most common osteotomy used for mild-to-moderate bunion deformities is the Austin, or chevron bunionectomy. In fact, in their original description of the procedure, Austin and Leventen[1] described the 60° V-shaped osteotomy being stabilized with only manual impaction. Despite this, most surgeons today would not take the risk of capital fragment displacement, which may likely occur with weight bearing. The simplest method of inserting a K-wire for fixation of the Austin bunionectomy is from dorsal-proximal-medial at the metatarsal, across the plantar arm of the osteotomy, and into the capital fragment plantarly.[6] One should take caution not to penetrate into the joint by distracting the joint and directly visualizing the metatarsal head. One downfall of K-wire fixation is backing out of the wire. This causes instability across the osteotomy site, and irritation underneath the skin. One mode of avoiding this is by using a locking technique. A small segment of wire is left prominent and is then rotated into a dorsal position on top of the metatarsal shaft. The wire is bent at an acute angle and is forced into the dorsal cortex. This creates more stability and prevents the K-wire from backing out because of the bending moment being transferred to the part of the K-wire that is inside the metatarsal head.[6] However, some authors argue that this technique actually results in a loss of compression with more reliance on the stability of the osteotomy than on the K-wire. In addition, there is still possibility of the K-wire becoming too prominent and causing symptoms from skin irritation.[7] Camasta[7] describes a technique in which a threaded 0.062 K-wire is used across the osteotomy site and then bent across a freer elevator to sit completely flush with the dorsal cortex. A second wire may be used in parallel fashion to the first if motion is still noted. Wire back out is extremely rare because of the threaded tip and therefore skin irritation and the need for removal are virtually obsolete. Coughlin[8] describes a technique in which the Kirschner wire is inserted percutaneously and removed in the office at 3 to 4 weeks. The patient is not allowed to begin full weight bearing in a surgical shoe until about 4 weeks and a weight-bearing cast may need to be applied if the osteotomy is not healing in a timely manner. This is a clear deterrent to many patients and surgeons because immediate weight bearing is possible with other forms of fixation.

Kirschner wires may even be an appropriate fixation option for fusions of the first ray. Specifically, in cases of severe osteoporosis and even rheumatoid arthritis, this may be the preferred fixation method. Although the position of the fusion is of the utmost importance to the final success of the surgery, the fixation method used may contribute to the stability of the fusion site and healing time. The key to ensuring bony consolidation with wire fixation is to make certain that satisfactory apposition between the two joint surfaces has occurred.[9]

Many different constructs have been described when using K-wires or even Steinman pins in the fixation of first metatarsophalangeal joint fusions. One of the most common techniques used is an intramedullary technique with two or three wires placed across the interphalangeal and metatarsophalangeal joints. This may prove useful when either a simultaneous hallux interphalangeal joint fusion is warranted, or even if a hallux extensus is present and correction with maintenance of alignment is desired.[9] However, fixation through an otherwise healthy interphalangeal joint may lead to arthritic changes and pain at the joint. Rotational instability can be avoided by redirecting a wire in an oblique fashion; if the surgeon prefers to avoid insertion of the K-wires through the interphalangeal joint, a cross K-wire technique may be implemented.[9] It is without a doubt that the most ideal postoperative course for a procedure of this nature is strict non–weight bearing. Nonetheless, some authors have described successful first metatarsophalangeal joint fusion with fixation using three 0.062 K-wires following immediate weight bearing in a surgical shoe padded with felt or cork extending from the heal to just distal to the digital sulcus.[10]

A combination of K-wire fixation and cerclage wiring to create a tension band technique for fusion of the first metatarsophalangeal joint has also been described.[11] This, again, is a feasible option for patients with poor bone stock.

STAPLE FIXATION

Although not as commonly used as some other more rigid fixation techniques, staple fixation can be a useful tool in hallux valgus surgery. The ability to provide some additional compression as opposed to K-wires, and the more low profile nature of the staple compared with a larger plate, makes staple fixation appealing to some surgeons. For staples to be effective, the cortical bone should not exceed 2 to 3 mm in thickness. If the cortical bone is thicker, predrilling is necessary. If this is not performed, there is a risk of cortical fracture or incomplete seating of the staple.[2] Studies have found that the shape of the staple legs does actually affect the pullout strength of the staple. The most secure shape was noted to be the curvilinear square, followed by a square configuration. The weakest configuration was that of a triangle.[2] To attain the greatest amount of compression from staple fixation, the legs should be oriented at 10° outward from vertical.[2]

In more recent years, the memory compression staple has become a popular choice for staple fixation. These staples are made out of a nickel titanium alloy. At low temperatures, the material is flexible and can be easily manipulated. However, at higher temperatures, such as those found in the body, the alloy reverts back to its original shape. As a result, when the staple is taken out of its frozen packaging the two legs are parallel to each other. When placed into the bone, the two arms move toward each other and create a dynamic compression effect.[12] One of the most powerful uses of staple fixation is for epiphysiodesis in treatment of juvenile hallux valgus. In this procedure, the staple is placed on the lateral aspect of the metatarsal to stall growth and correct the deformity.

Staples may be used for fixation of Akin osteotomies but the surgeon must be aware of a few key points (**Fig. 3**). First, the contour of the proximal phalanx may cause the staple not to sit completely flush with the bone and can result in underlying skin irritation. Second, especially in a small patient, caution must be taken not to violate the joint with the leg of the staple. In addition, the bone at the phalanx may be softer with a thinner cortical layer and there is risk of fracture with insertion of the staple. Nevertheless, if appropriately used, staple fixation may be a simple method to fixating a proximal phalanx osteotomy.

Although not as readily implemented, staples may be used for osteotomies and fusions in the first ray. Most often, they are used as adjunct fixation if the primary form of fixation proves to be insufficient. Some have described using a single staple technique for fixation of an Austin bunionectomy. Recommendations are for insertion of the staple from proximal-dorsal to plantar-distal. The stated advantages of using this form of fixation include the ability to perform the procedure with minimal dissection and, more importantly, the ability for the staple to afford some plantar compression. This is important when early weight bearing is desired. It has been shown that with ground reactive forces, the dorsal surface of the osteotomy tends to compress, while gapping occurs plantarly.[13]

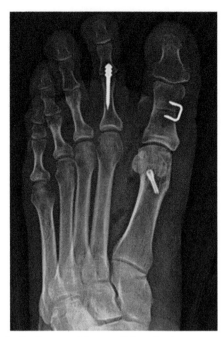

Fig. 3. Example of staple fixation used for an Akin osteotomy.

Reports of successful fusion of the first metatarsophalangeal joint with compression staples have also been found. Vanore[14] describes various cases of first metatarsophalangeal joint arthrodesis with one dorsal to plantar staple across the fusion site. The one caveat in using this technique is that it may be required to shorten the distal arm of the staple to accommodate for the thinner proximal phalanx. If further fixation is desired, an additional staple inserted from medial to lateral can be used. This demonstrates that other valid alternatives for use of plates and screws exist, and that these alternatives can provide rigid internal fixation, which is comparable with that of other more current forms of fixation.[14]

Staple use for the Lapidus procedure is also an option. In fact, in studying various fixation devices for first tarsometatarsal fusions in sawbones, Chang and coworkers[15] found that memory staples are beneficial in providing true dynamic compression across the fusion site. They describe a construct similar to that of the first metatarsophalangeal joint fusion with one staple placed dorsally and the other medially.[15]

SCREW FIXATION

By far the most prevalent form of fixation used in foot and ankle surgery is that of screw fixation. Screws provide stability by producing interfragmentary compression across an osteotomy or fusion site. The Association for the Study of Internal Fixation emphasizes the importance of stable internal fixation to allow for earlier return to function. Various types of screws exist. Cortical screws have threads along the entire length of the shaft. These screws can be used in bunion correction surgery if proper lag technique is followed and adequate cortical bone is available. Cancellous screws have a larger thread-to-core ratio, and a larger pitch for a more adequate bite into cancellous bone. Cancellous screws are slightly weaker than cortical screws. In more recent years, cannulated screws have become a popular screw choice for many surgeons. A K-wire is used for provisional fixation and the screw is then placed over the wire for insertion. Most companies create cannulated screws that are self-drilling and self-tapping, which can reduce operating room time. In addition, the cannulated system is helpful when attempting to insert a screw in an oblique fashion, because noncannu-lated screws have a tendency to skive the far cortex. Although most claim that pull out strength of cannulated screws is lower than their solid counterparts, some studies have shown the exact opposite in smaller-diameter screw sizes.[16] Headless screws are also implemented frequently to decrease skin irritation and therefore screw removal. Some manufactures have also begun to more readily use variations of vari-able pitch, Herbert-like screws to increase compressive forces across the osteotomy site.

Osteotomies are the ideal procedures for screw fixation. The Akin osteotomy can be modified to accommodate for screw insertion (**Fig. 4**). The osteotomy must be oriented obliquely to allow for screw placement perpendicular to the osteotomy site. Screw size may vary from 2 to 2.7 mm depending on screw manufacturer and size of the patient. Caution to maintain the hinge should be taken even more critically, because the oblique cut is not as stable as the transverse cut described earlier. If the hinge is compromised, it is suggested that a secondary point of fixation be inserted for further stability.

It is without question that screw fixation for osteotomies of the first metatarsal have become routine practice for most surgeons. The preference for screw fixation and orientation in distal osteotomies depends on the type of osteotomy performed. The classic chevron bunionectomy requires a screw to be placed from proximal to distal into the metatarsal head. Because the screw does not engage cortical bone, in

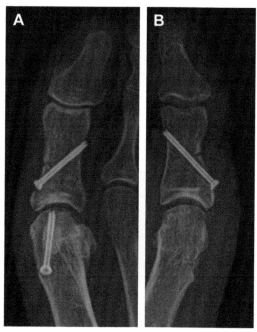

Fig. 4. (A, B) Two examples of an Akin osteotomy fixated with single screw. Note the obliq-uity of the osteotomy to accommodate for screw insertion.

addition to the fact that the screw is being placed into an area that is difficult to visualize, a cannulated screw is recommended (**Fig. 5**). Some have even described screw orientation from distal-dorsal to proximal-plantar. However, a higher rate of capital fragment displacement has been found with this construct.[17] Murphy and colleagues[17] advocate a technique combining both forms of fixation. Using two 3-mm headless cannulated screws in crossed fashion allowed for slightly faster healing time in their study patients. In addition, fewer incidences of displacement occurred compared with the group that was fixated with only a distal to proximal screw.

Contrary to the fixation of the Austin bunionectomy, cortical screws are warranted for fixation of long dorsal and plantar arm cuts. It is crucial that the screws be oriented perpendicular to the osteotomy site (**Fig. 6**). Headless and cannulated screws are also options if the surgeon so prefers. If one elects to perform a long plantar arm osteotomy, the most distal screw can be modified to be inserted more into the cancellous portion of the metatarsal head as in the fixation for the Austin bunionectomy (**Fig. 7**). Fixation of the distal head and metatarsal shaft osteotomies with proper screw configuration creates a stable construct that can allow the patient to bear weight in protective shoe gear immediately postoperatively.

Proximal metatarsal osteotomies are also very conducive to screw fixation. For example, the ideal fixation construct for closing base wedge osteotomies is with two cancellous or cortical screws. The first screw is oriented perpendicular to the long axis of the bone. This is known as the anchor screw. Subsequently, the compression screw is inserted perpendicular to the osteotomy. Although screw fixation is used, the patient is still kept non–weight bearing for about 6 weeks.

Screw fixation is also an excellent choice for fusions. Single screw fixation for first metatarsophalangeal joint fusions is a possibility; however, bone quality must be excellent for proper compression to be achieved. The screw may be placed from the medial aspect of the proximal phalanx and into the lateral aspect of the metatarsal head. K-wires can be added to this construct to prevent rotational stresses.[9] A more

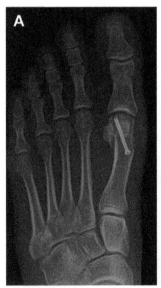
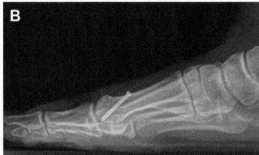

Fig. 5. (*A, B*) Anteroposterior and lateral views of long plantar arm osteotomy fixated with a single screw.

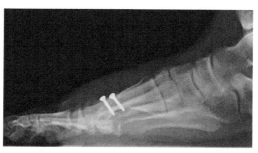

Fig. 6. Long dorsal arm osteotomy fixated with two screws perpendicular to the osteotomy site.

accepted approach is that of the two crossed screw technique (**Fig. 8**). Here, the cannulated systems provide ease of insertion and confirmation of proper screw placement. As with any screw insertion, it is imperative that the threads cross the fusion site to attain sufficient compression. To avoid prominence of the screws and the need for removal, the surgeon should attempt to place the screws at the metaphyseal flare of the proximal phalanx and metatarsal. Additionally, appropriate countersinking should be performed to minimize screw head protrusion.[9]

Crossed screw technique is also a popular construct for fixation of first metatarsal cuneiform joint fusions and is also facilitated by use of cannulated screws (**Fig. 9**). Proper screw placement is important for the success of the procedure. The key screw is oriented from distal dorsal over the metatarsal and is inserted into the plantar aspect of the cuneiform. One should attempt to place the screw as parallel as possible to the weight-bearing surface of the foot. The second screw may either be inserted from the dorsal aspect of the cuneiform and into the plantar aspect of the first metatarsal base, or it can be oriented from the plantar-medial aspect of the first metatarsal and into the dorsal-lateral aspect of the cuneiform. Supplemental fixation with other screws or pins

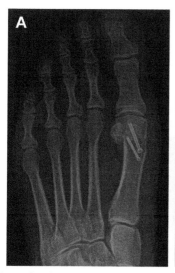
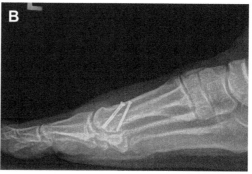

Fig. 7. (A, B) Anteroposterior and lateral views of a long plantar arm osteotomy fixated with two cannulated screws.

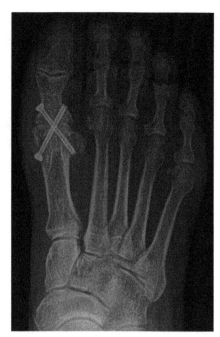

Fig. 8. First metatarsophalangeal joint fusion with two crossed screw technique.

may always be added as needed depending on bone quality and severity of deformity. Some modifications have been described that allow the patient to bear weight in protective immobilization boot immediately after surgery. Basile and coworkers[18] implement a technique in which a 0.062 K-wire is inserted percutaneously from the medial aspect of the first metatarsal at the level of the midshaft and through both cortices of

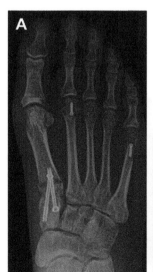

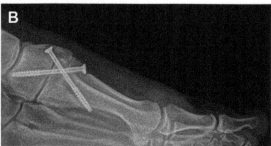

Fig. 9. (*A, B*) Lapidus bunionectomy fixated with two crossed screws.

the second metatarsal. The wire is then removed about 3 months postoperatively. The author believes that this wire neutralizes the torque at the fusion site by reducing the level arm effect, thereby allowing weight bearing without damage to the arthrodesis.

PLATE FIXATION

Many different plate types exist and they can be used in various ways. Low-profile plates work best because plates are either placed dorsally or medially where little subcutaneous fat exists to protect from skin irritation. Conventional stainless steel plates provide increased rigidity and should therefore be used in situations that require a rigid fixation construct. Still, titanium plates are often a good option because titanium is less stiff than stainless steel and therefore decreases the risk of stress shielding.[9] Although most plates in the first ray are used for fusions, many manufacturers have now created specialty wedge plates that can be used for other procedures, such as opening base wedges.

Locking plates have recently come into favor for first metatarsophalangeal joint and first metatarsocuneiform joint fusions (**Figs. 10** and **11**). Locking plates are particularly useful in patients with soft, osteopenic bone. Conventional plates require adequate purchase of screws to obtain compression between the plate and cortical bone and are therefore not indicated in patients with poor bone stock. On the contrary, locking plates do not require compression of the plate directly onto the bone to provide stability. The locking mechanism also decreases toggle and therefore backing out of the screw is minimized.[19] In most scenarios, a combination of locking and nonlocking screws is used to fixate the plate. The nonlocking screws are helpful in areas of irregular contour to allow the plate to sit flush with the bone.

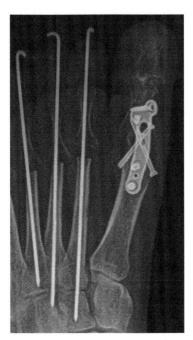

Fig. 10. Example of first metatarsophalangeal joint fusion fixated with two crossed screws supplemented with dorsal locking plate.

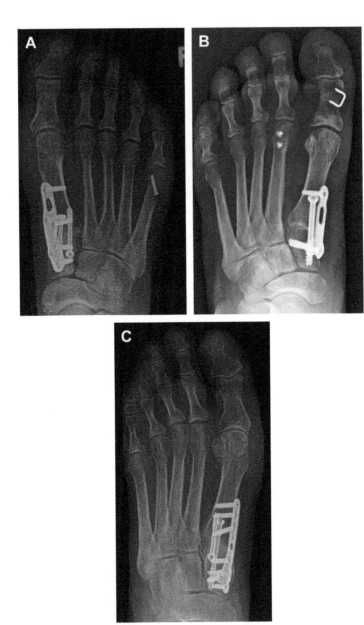

Fig. 11. (*A–C*) Various configurations of screw and locking plate constructs for first metatarsocuneiform joint fusions.

An interfragmentary screw is usually used along with the plate fixation to increase the level of compression across the fusion site. Nevertheless, most plates now have an added hole for placement of an eccentric screw, which can afford compression directly through the plate. Hyer and colleagues[20] compared four different plating constructs and evaluated their effect on union in first metatarsophalangeal joint fusions. Although a locked plate with lag screw configuration resulted in a slightly increased rate of union compared with a locked plate without a lag screw and a static plate with and without a lag screw, this was not statistically significant.[20] It should be noted that all patients were allowed weight bearing in a tall walking boot after 1 week of immobilization in a splint.

As the trend for early weight bearing continues, many studies have been performed comparing plate fixation with crossed screw fixation in first metatarsophalangeal and metatarsocuneiform fusions. In comparing the biomechanics in locking versus non-locking plates in cadaveric models, Hunt and coworkers[21] found locking plates to result in significantly less plantar gapping with fatigue endurance testing, and greater stiffness in load-to-failure testing. Doty and coworkers[22] relate good results with im-mediate protected, partial weight bearing following first metatarsophalangeal joint fusion with a locking plate and plantar screw. Although results for early weight bearing with locking plates are promising, some studies still present controversy. In a clinical study, Hunt and coworkers[23] found a slightly higher rate of nonunion when using a locked titanium plate versus a nonlocked stainless steel plate in first metatarsophalan-geal joint fusions with early weight bearing.

Positive outcomes have been described with Lapidus fusion. Saxena and co-workers[24] found no difference in union rates of the Lapidus procedure when comparing fixation with two crossed screws and locking plate with a plantar lag screw. Interestingly, the patients who received fixation with the locking plate began weight bearing at 4 weeks versus 6 weeks in the crossed screw cohort with no increase in complication rate.[24] Another study evaluating the Lapidus arthrodesis with a dorso-medial locking plate and lag screw related a 0% nonunion rate with return to ambula-tion in 2 weeks.[25] Nevertheless, others advocate fixation with a plantar plate and interfragmentary screw and argue that a plantar plate best negates ground reactive forces and elevation of the metatarsal.[26]

SUMMARY

No matter the fixation method a surgeon elects, if proper technique is implemented for the appropriate procedure, a good result should be expected. One should also keep in mind the postoperative course differs based on the fixation construct. Improper management after surgery with nonrigid, unstable fixation methods can lead to detrimental outcomes for the patient. The surgeon should be conscious of all fixation options available for hallux valgus correction and use each appropriately and when indicated.

REFERENCES

1. Austin DW, Leventen EO. A new osteotomy for hallux valgus: a horizontally directed "V" displacement osteotomy of the metatarsal head for hallux valgus and primus varus. Clin Orthop 1981;157:25–30.
2. Ray RG, et al. Methods of osseous fixation. In: Banks AS, Downey MS, Martin DE, et al, editors. McGlamry's comprehensive textbook of foot and ankle surgery. 3rd edition. Philadelphia: Lippincott Williams and Wilkins; 2001. p. 65–106.
3. Burns AE. Surgical procedures of the hallux. In: Banks AS, Downey MS, Martin DE, et al, editors. McGlamry's comprehensive textbook of foot and ankle surgery. 3rd edition. Philadelphia: Lippincott Williams and Wilkins; 2001. p. 639–54.
4. Chacon Y, Fallat LM, Dau N, et al. Biomechanical comparison of internal fixation techniques for the Akin osteotomy of the proximal phalanx. J Foot Ankle Surg 2012;51:561–5.
5. Zelen CM, Yound NJ. Alternative methods in fixation for capital osteotomies in hallux valgus surgery. Clin Podiatr Med Surg 2013;30:295–306.

6. Chang TJ. Distal metaphyseal osteotomies in hallux abducto valgus surgery. In: Banks AS, Downey MS, Martin DE, et al, editors. McGlamry's comprehensive textbook of foot and ankle surgery. 3rd edition. Philadelphia: Lippincott Williams and Wilkins; 2001. p. 505–27.

7. Camasta CA. Threaded Kirschner-wire fixation of the Austin bunionectomy: simplified technique. Podiatry Institute Update 2008;61–4 chapter 13.

8. Coughlin MJ. Hallux valgus. J Bone Joint Surg Am 1996;78:932–66.

9. Yu GV, Shook JE. Arthrodesis of the first metatarsophalangeal joint. In: Banks AS, Downey MS, Martin DE, et al, editors. McGlamry's comprehensive textbook of foot and ankle surgery. 3rd edition. Philadelphia: Lippincott Williams and Wilkins; 2001. p. 581–607.

10. Mah CD, Banks A. Immediate weightbearing following first MPJ fusion with Kirschner-wire fixation. Podiatry Institute Update 2007;21:111–4.

11. Malay DS. Tension band wire fixation of the first metatarsal phalangeal arthrodesis. Podiatry Institute Update 1993;394–7.

12. Choudhary RK, Theruvil B, Taylor GR, et al. First metatarsophalangeal joint arthrodesis: a new technique of internal fixation by using memory compression staples. J Foot Ankle Surg 2004;43(5):312–7.

13. Boberg JS, Oldani T, Grieder R. Austin bunionectomy with compression staple fixation. Podiatry Institute Update 2007;19:105–6.

14. Vanore JV. First metatarsophalangeal joint fusion with minimal fixation. Podiatry Institute Update 2010;36:215–24.

15. Chang TJ, Overley BD, Pancrantz D. An in vitro comparative study of screw and nitinol staple compression: a model showing active dynamic compression. Podiatry Institute Update 2008;32:178–84.

16. Kissel CG, Freidersdorf SC, Foltz DS, et al. Comparison of pullout strength of small-diameter cannulated and solid-core screws. J Foot Ankle Surg 2003; 42(6):334–8.

17. Murphy RM, Fallat LM, Kish JP. Axial loading screw fixation for chevron type osteotomies of the distal first metatarsal: a retrospective outcomes analysis. J Foot Ankle Surg 2013;53(1):52–4.

18. Basile P, Cook EA, Cook JJ. Immediate weight bearing following modified lapidus arthrodesis. J Foot Ankle Surg 2010;49:459–64.

19. Kim T, Ayturk UM, Haskell A, et al. Fixation of osteoporotic distal fibula fractures: a biomechanical comparison of locking versus conventional plates. J Foot Ankle Surg 2007;46(1):2–6.

20. Hyer CF, Scott RT, Swiatek M. A retrospective comparison of four plate constructs for first metatarsophalangeal joint fusion: static plate with lag screw, locked plate, and locked plate with lag screw. J Foot Ankle Surg 2012;51:285–7.

21. Hunt KJ, Barr CR, Lindsey DP, et al. Locked versus nonlocked plate fixation for first metatarsophalangeal arthrodesis: a biomechanical investigation. Foot Ankle Int 2012;33:984–90.

22. Doty J, Coughlin M, Hirose C, et al. Hallux metatarsophalangeal joint arthrodesis with hybrid locking plate and a plantar neutralization screw: a prospective study. Foot Ankle Int 2013;34(11):1535–40.

23. Hunt KJ, Ellington JK, Anderson RB, et al. Locked versus nonlocked plate fixation for hallux MTP arthrodesis. Foot Ankle Int 2011;32(7):704–9.

24. Saxena A, Nguyen A, Nelsen E. Lapidus bunionectomy: early evaluation of crossed lag screws versus locking plate with plantar lag screw. J Foot Ankle Surg 2009;48(2):170–9.

25. Sorensen MD, Hyer CF, Berlet GC. Results of lapidus arthrodesis and locked plating with early weight bearing. Foot Ankle Spec 2009;2:227–33.
26. Gutteck N, Wohlrab D, Zeh A, et al. Comparative study of lapidus bunionectomy using different osteosynthesis methods. Foot Ankle Surg 2013;19:218–21.

First Metatarsophalangeal Joint Arthrodesis in the Treatment of Hallux Valgus

J. Braxton Little, DPM

KEYWORDS

- Hallux valgus • Arthrodesis • First metatarsophalangeal joint • Fusion

KEY POINTS

- First metatarsal phalangeal joint (MPJ) arthrodesis has long been a reliable procedure in the armamentarium of the foot and ankle surgeon.
- The primary goal of first MPJ fusion should be to reduce/eliminate pain associated with the structural and functional changes related to the attendant pathology.
- Recent advances in fixation technique, coupled with early weight bearing and reliable, predictable, outcome make first MPJ an attractive alternative for the foot and ankle surgeon.

First metatarsal phalangeal joint (MPJ) arthrodesis has long been a reliable procedure in the armamentarium of the foot and ankle surgeon. First described over 100 years ago, the procedure has remained a go-to in salvage of first MPJ pathology.

End-stage degenerative disease has been the most common entity leading to arthrodesis of the first MPJ. Hallux varus, failed previous surgery (cheilectomy, implant arthroplasty), trauma, infection, rheumatoid arthritis, and neuromuscular disorders are but a few of the conditions amenable to first MPJ fusion. Moderate-to-severe hallux valgus with degenerative changes deemed contraindicated for a joint preservation procedure also falls into this category. When other procedures have previously failed or are simply not indicated, fusion can be an acceptable alternative for the surgeon in the treatment of hallux valgus with associated moderate-to-severe increase in first intermetatarsal angle.

In a study by Sung and colleagues,[1] it was shown that first MPJ arthrodesis could reduce a severe preoperative IM by an average of 6.7°. In moderate deformities, performing a first MPJ arthrodesis can reduce the preoperative inter-metatarsal angle (IM) by an average of 4.3°. Similarly, Cronin and colleagues[2] found mean change in intermetatarsal angle of 8.22°. In these studies, as the preoperative IM angle increased,

Private Practice, University Foot and Ankle Institute, 2121 Wilshire Boulevard, Santa Monica, CA 90403, USA
E-mail address: jbl827@aol.com

Clin Podiatr Med Surg 31 (2014) 281–289
http://dx.doi.org/10.1016/j.cpm.2013.12.009
0891-8422/14/$ – see front matter © 2014 Elsevier Inc. All rights reserved.

so did the corresponding degree of reduction achieved with the fusion. Similarly, significant reduction was noted in the hallux abductus angle also. Dayton, LoPiccolo, and Kiley, based on similar findings in their study, came to the now accepted finding that osteotomy is generally not needed to address high IM angles when fusing the first MPJ.[3]

Severe IM and Hallux abductus (HA) angles as well as rotational deformities can be reduced and maintained with first MPJ fusion. This has led to better acceptance of first MPJ arthrodesis in treating this patient population.

The primary goal of first MPJ fusion should be to reduce/eliminate pain associated with the structural and functional changes related to the attendant pathology. As a result, there may be improvement in overall functional outcome also. Multiple authors have shown good-to-excellent results without significant restriction in activity. They attribute the excellent outcomes of arthrodesis to multiple factors:

1. Permanent correction with low likelihood of recurrence
2. Advantageous in patients with severe arthrosis, laxity and/or contracture
3. Preserves weight-bearing function better than resection arthroplasty or implant arthroplasty
4. Medial column stability is improved, leading to reduction of pain associated with lesser metatarsalgia[3,4]

In their recent article comparing hemi implant arthroplasty, total joint replacement and first MPJ arthrodesis, Erdil and colleagues[5] found that at final follow-up, functional assessment using the AOFAS-HMI (American Orthopedic Foot and Ankle Society-Hallux Metatarsophalangeal-Interphalangeal) scoring system was similar when comparing all 3 procedures. However, the visual analog scale (VAS) scores were much better with arthrodesis. In his review of the literature, Brewster found that arthrodesis achieved better functional outcomes than total joint replacement.[6]

Once the determination has been made to proceed with arthrodesis, there are critical components that are key in the successful outcome of the procedure. These are: joint preparation, position of arthrodesis, method of fixation, and postoperative management.

JOINT PREPARATION

Historically, the joint was often prepared by squaring off the opposing joint surfaces of the phalanx and metatarsal head to create a broad, flat, end-to-end fusion. Although shown to be a more stable construct, this technique is prone to excessive shortening of the first ray and inherently prevents the surgeon from being able to easily manipulate the fusion site in all 3 planes to achieve optimal positioning. Joint contour preservation techniques ameliorate these issues. In first MPJ arthrodesis, the result of joint preparation is a cone-and-cup (ball-and-socket) construct, in which the convexity of the first metatarsal head and the concavity of the base of the proximal phalanx are maintained.

A standard dorsomedial approach is used to gain access to the joint. Excessive stripping of soft tissue from the first metatarsal head and neck area is to be avoided (**Figs. 1** and **2**). Joint preparation begins by removing any surrounding periarticular bony abnormalities with a rongeur and bur. Soft tissue and the sesamoids are dealt with according to specific attendant pathology and surgeon preference. Attention is then directed to the opposing joint surfaces.

The goal in appropriate joint preparation is to remove any remaining diseased cartilage and its corresponding subchondral bone. Johnson and colleagues[7] showed that curettage technique alone often left a barrier of subchondral bone that could act as an impediment to successful fusion. Subchondral drilling has been advocated as

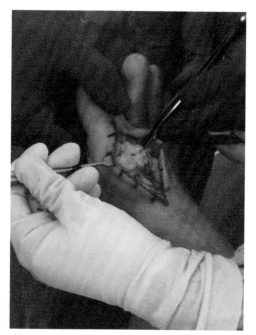

Fig. 1. Standard dorsomedial approach to joint.

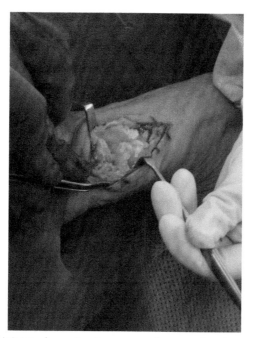

Fig. 2. Exposure of joint surfaces showing severe degenerative changes and periarticular osteophytes.

a means to perforate the subchondral plate and expose bleeding bone to improve the migration of osseous cells to the site.[8,9] However, based on the findings of Johnson and colleagues,[7] this may leave a significant barrier to fusion. Shingling, or fish scaling, is another method used in joint surface preparation. Using an osteotome and mallet, the subchondral plate is fenestrated in multiple planes to morselize the plate and expose bleeding cancellous bone. As mentioned previously, this technique may leave a barrier of subchondral bone that can perhaps lead to a delayed union or nonunion. A thin periarticular rim of the plate is left intact for stability.

Reaming systems have been developed to assist in joint preparation. These systems can be used manually or with power (**Figs. 3** and **4**). Although excellent at exposing cancellous subchondral bone, care must be taken to avoid excess bone resection that can occur easily when used with power instrumentation. In the author's institution, surgeons generally use a power reaming system to prepare the opposing joint surfaces. A rongeur is used to remove remaining osteophytes and remodel the periarticular margins (**Fig. 5**). Joint preparation is completed with subchondral drilling (**Fig. 6**).

POSITION OF ARTHRODESIS

As mentioned previously, the ball-and-socket construct allows the surgeon to easily manipulate the joint into position for fusion while preventing excess bone removal. A flat, rigid surface such as the top of an instrument tray is used to load the foot in a slightly pronated position. It is important to load the foot to more closely mimic the inclination angle of the first metatarsal while weight bearing. The hallux is then placed in position in the transverse plane roughly parallel to the position of the second toe. This translates into a position somewhere between 10° and 15° of abduction.

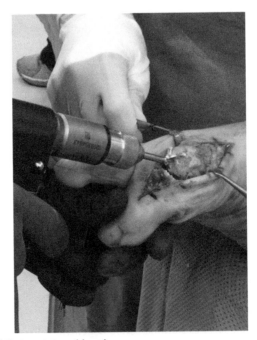

Fig. 3. Reaming of first metatarsal head.

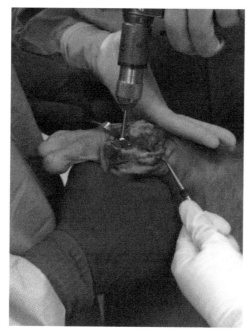

Fig. 4. Reaming of proximal phalanx base.

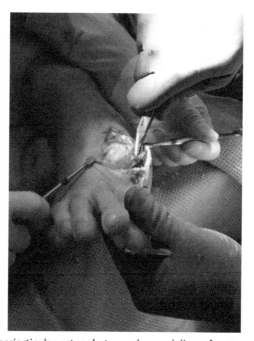

Fig. 5. Removal of periarticular osteophytes and remodeling of metatarsal head.

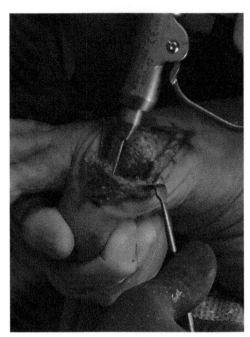

Fig. 6. Subchondral drilling with k-wire. Note adequate preparation of metatarsal head with complete removal of subchondral bone.

Sagittal plane alignment is achieved by sliding the end of the fifth finger (pinky finger) under the hallux just to a point where it contacts the level of the hallux interphalangeal joint (IPJ) at the head of the proximal phalanx. Care should be taken not to mistake the often-attendant hallux IPJ hyperextension as MPJ dorsiflexion. This translates into roughly 15° to 25° of dorsiflexion. Coughlin reported an increase in prevalence of hallux IPJ arthritis in joints fused at less than 20°.[10] Tanabe and colleagues,[11] in their study of sagittal plane alignment after first MPJ fusion, found that general agreement of the sagittal angle for the first MPJ varies and that the optimal alignment of the first MPJ is still controversial. Care should be taken to avoid any frontal plane rotation. The hallux is then fixated in a corrected position based on surgeon preference.

METHOD OF FIXATION

The general tenet of rigid compression for arthrodesis applies to the first MPJ as it does in other arthrodesis sites. Multiple techniques have been described in the literature. A thorough review of the literature on fixation options beyond the scope of this paper is available in Joseph Treadwell's article in *Clinics in Podiatric Medicine and Surgery*.[12]

Buranosky and colleagues,[13] in their study on cadaveric stress testing, found that a dorsal 6-hole plate with single lag screw was a stronger construct than 2 crossed screws. Similarly, Politi and colleagues,[14] using synthetic bone models, found that a dorsal plate and single lag screw provided a more stable construct than single lag screw, dorsal plate alone, and crossed k-wires. However, large group prospective in vivo studies are needed to determine how these findings translate to the patient population undergoing first MPJ arthrodesis. The issue of a stable construct has become more important as the move toward early weight bearing in first MPJ fusion has gained popularity.

POSTOPERATIVE MANAGEMENT

Historically, patients who underwent first MPJ fusion were maintained on strict non-weight bearing for an average of 6 weeks followed by gradual return to shoe gear and activities. Postoperative splinting included methods such as: Jones compression dressings, rigid posterior splints, rigid below the knee casts, removable cast boots, and surgical shoes. It was generally accepted that early weight bearing would lead to increased incidence of nonunion.

However, as shown in Dayton and McCall's retrospective review, this may not be the case. They had a 100% union rate in 47 fusions in which patients were allowed to bear weight in a surgical shoe within the first week.[15] Mah and Banks concluded that their findings agreed with many previous authors who found acceptable union rates associated with early weight bearing.[16] In perhaps the largest retrospective study to date, Roukis, Meusnier, and Augoyard found early weight bearing in a protective shoe with their fixation construct showed lower incidence of nonunion when compared with other studies.[17]

The difficulty for the practitioner lies in the fact that the definition of early weight bearing and the type of fixation construct used varies greatly between articles. Certainly, the prospect of early weight bearing makes the procedure more attractive to patients and surgeons. It also has practical implications. Muscle atrophy and joint stiffness perhaps would be minimized on the operative side. Contralateral limb stress, back stress, and upper extremity problems associated with crutches would also be minimized. So, too, would the potential for falls in the elderly or compromised patient.

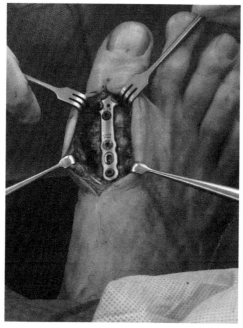

Fig. 7. Plate and crossed screw fixation.

Potential complications specific to this procedure include: delayed union, malunion, nonunion, pseudoarthrosis, malposition of hallux, lesser metatarsalgia, and hallux IPJ arthritis.

Currently, at the University Foot and Ankle Institute, a dorsal plate with a single lag screw or crossed screw configuration across the joint in the transverse plane is used (**Fig. 7**). Patients are immobilized nonweight bearing in a below-the-knee fiberglass cast for 2 weeks followed by transition to a cast boot. Heel weight bearing is encouraged from weeks 2 through 4 postoperatively. Full weight bearing in the boot is allowed in weeks 4 through 6 and then transition to a stiff-soled athletic shoe as tolerated.

In conclusion, first MPJ fusion as a stand alone in the treatment of moderate-to-severe hallux valgus with degenerative changes has been shown to be an excellent alternative to joint arthroplasty with or without implants. Recent advances in fixation technique, coupled with early weight bearing and reliable, predictable, outcome, makes the procedure an attractive alternative for the foot and ankle surgeon.

REFERENCES

1. Sung W, Kluesner AJ, Irrgang J, et al. Radiographic outcomes following primary arthrodesis of the first metatarsophalangeal joint in hallux abductovalgus deformity. J Foot Ankle Surg 2010;49(5):446–51.
2. Cronin JJ, Limbers JP, Kutty S, et al. Intermetatarsal angle after first metatarsophalangeal arthrodesis for hallux valgus. Foot Ankle Int 2006;27(2):104–9.
3. Dayton P, Lopiccolo J, Kiley J. Reduction of the intermetatarsal angle after first metatarsophalangeal joint arthrodesis in patients with moderate and severe metatarsus primus adductus. J Foot Ankle Surg 2002;41:316–9.
4. Coughlin MJ, Grebing BR, Jones CP. Arthrodesis of the first metatarsophalangeal joint for idiopathic hallux valgus: intermediate results. Foot Ankle Int 2005;26:783–92.
5. Erdil M, Elmadağ NM, Polat G, et al. Comparison of arthrodesis, resurfacing hemiarthroplasty, and total joint replacement in the treatment of advanced hallux rigidus. J Foot Ankle Surg 2013;52(5):588–93.
6. Brewster M. Does total joint replacement or arthrodesis of the first metatarsophalangeal joint yield better functional results? A systematic review of the literature. J Foot Ankle Surg 2010;49:546–52.
7. Johnson JT, Schuberth JM, Thornton SD, et al. Joint curettage arthrodesis technique in the foot: a histological analysis. J Foot Ankle Surg 2009;48(5):558–64.
8. Yu GV. The curettage technique for major rearfoot fusions. In: Camasta CA, Vickers NS, Ruch JA, editors. The Podiatry Institute reconstructive surgery of the foot and leg, Update '93. Tucker (GA): Podiatry Institute; 1993. p. 260–7.
9. Coetzee JC, Wickum D. The Lapidus procedure: a prospective cohort outcome study. Foot Ankle Int 2004;25:526–31.
10. Coughlin MJ. Rheumatoid forefoot reconstruction: a long-term follow-up study. J Bone Joint Surg Am 2000;82:322–41.
11. Tanabe A, Majima T, Onodera T, et al. Sagittal alignment of the first metatarsophalangeal joint after arthrodesis for rheumatoid forefoot deformity. J Foot Ankle Surg 2013;52(3):343–7.
12. Treadwell JR. First metatarsophalangeal joint arthrodesis; what is the best fixation option? A critical review of the literature. Clin Podiatr Med Surg 2013;30:327–49.
13. Buranosky DJ, Taylor DT, Sage RA, et al. First metatarsophalangeal joint arthrodesis: quantitative mechanical testing of six-hole dorsal plate versus crossed screw fixation in cadaveric specimens. J Foot Ankle Surg 2001;40:208–13.

14. Politi J, Hayes J, Njus G, et al. First metatarsal-phalangeal joint arthrodesis: a biomechanical assessment of stability. Foot Ankle Int 2003;24:332–7.
15. Dayton P, McCall A. Early weightbearing after first metatarsophalangeal joint arthrodesis: a retrospective observational case analysis. J Foot Ankle Surg 2004;43:156–9.
16. Mah CD, Banks AS. Immediate weight bearing following first metatarsophalangeal joint fusion with Kirschner wire fixation. J Foot Ankle Surg 2009;48:3–8.
17. Roukis TS, Meusnier T, Augoyard M. Incidence of nonunion of first metatarsophalangeal joint arthrodesis for severe hallux valgus using crossed, flexible titanium intramedullary nails and a dorsal static staple with immediate weightbearing in female patients. J Foot Ankle Surg 2012;51(4):433–6.

Revision Hallux Valgus
Causes and Correction Options

Bob Baravarian, DPM[a],*, Rotem Ben-Ad, DPM[b]

KEYWORDS

- Hallux varus • Revision hallux valgus • Failed hallux valgus correction
- Avascular necrosis • Nonunion • Malunion • Bunion revision • Bunion reoccurrence

KEY POINTS

- Revision bunion surgery can be difficult and must be worked up thoroughly.
- Avascular necrosis can result in severe bone damage and limit potential options for revision surgery.
- The most common causes of revision surgery are reoccurrence, malunion, nonunion, and hallux varus.

CAUSES OF HALLUX VALGUS FAILURE

Hallux valgus failure has a multitude of causes. Too many potential causes exist to be discussed completely in this article, but the most common causes are addressed.

RECURRENCE

Recurrence of hallux valgus after surgical correction is undoubtedly a frustrating scenario for both patient and surgeon. Austin and colleagues[1] found a 10% recurrence rate on retrospective review of 300 Chevron osteotomies performed. A common theme among all recurrence was a preoperative hallux abductus angle greater than 35°, and an intermetatarsal angle of greater than 15°. Lagaay and colleagues[2] described a 5.56% reoperation rate in a retrospective analysis of Chevron osteotomies, with recurrence being the most common reason for return to the operating room. Many causes of recurrent hallux valgus deformity have been described, most of which involve inadequate patient selection and inadequate procedure selection, which can be catastrophic to the overall outcome for the patient. For example, performing a head osteotomy in a patient with a severe intermetatarsal angle may not

[a] UCLA Medical Center, Santa Monica/UCLA Medical Center and Orthopedic Hospital, University Foot and Ankle Institute, Los Angeles, CA, USA; [b] University Foot and Ankle Institute, Los Angeles, CA, USA
* Corresponding author.
E-mail address: BBaravarian@mednet.ucla.edu

Clin Podiatr Med Surg 31 (2014) 291–298
http://dx.doi.org/10.1016/j.cpm.2013.12.010
0891-8422/14/$ – see front matter © 2014 Elsevier Inc. All rights reserved.

afford proper correction. Even if soft tissue rebalancing with aggressive capsular reefing gives the impression of adequate correction, the risk of deformity return is high. Additionally, failure to recognize the need for supplementary procedures, such as an Akin, may lead to continued lateral deviation of the hallux with abnormal pull of the tendons about the first metatarsophalangeal joint. Inappropriate intraoperative technique is also a common cause of reoccurring hallux valgus. More specifically, insufficient lateral release with poor sesamoid realignment, improper repair of the medial capsule, inadequate repair of the intermetatarsal angle, or a deficiency in hardware fixation all may lead to deformity recurrence.[3] In addition, failure to address a hypermobile first ray can lead to an unfavorable outcome for patients with persistence of symptoms. Other causes that are less under surgeon control have also been described. For example, Okuda and colleagues[4] found that a more roundly shaped metatarsal head was more predisposed to postoperative hallux valgus recurrence when compared with a more angular metatarsal head. Through identifying this in the preoperative planning process, the surgeon can modify the procedure accordingly to prevent return of the bunion.

Procedures for revisional surgery can be divided into joint-sparing and joint-destructive procedures. If the deformity is still mild to moderate in nature and no severe arthritic changes are present, a joint-sparing procedure may still be an option.[5] The surgeon may consider another osteotomy either distally or proximally, a double osteotomy, or a Lapidus bunionectomy. In any case, capsulotendon rebalancing will most likely also be needed around the first metatarsophalangeal joint. Good results have been found with the use of a scarf osteotomy for revisional bunion surgery. One study demonstrated a mean American Orthopaedic Foot & Ankle Society (AOFAS) score improvement from 59 to 90, with a mean reduction in intermetatarsal angle from 13° to 4°.[6] Reoperation with a crescentic osteotomy has also been illustrated in the literature with good long-term outcomes.[5] Lim and Huntley[7] describe a 39-year-old woman previously treated with a Chevron osteotomy who presented with recurrence of her hallux valgus deformity. A proximal opening wedge was performed in combination with a short distal scarf osteotomy in which a medial closing wedge was used. Her 3-month postoperative visit showed both adequate clinical and radiographic outcomes.

The Lapidus arthrodesis is a reliable and reproducible procedure that is often used in secondary surgery for hallux valgus correction, especially if a significant amount of distal work has already been performed. The Lapidus procedure is a valid alternative if a severe intermetatarsal angle exists and first metatarsophalangeal joint salvage is desired. The procedure will also address any underlying hypermobility that may have been overlooked initially, and will provide overall stability to the medial column. Ellington and colleagues[8] performed a retrospective review of 32 feet treated with a Lapidus arthrodesis for recurrent hallux valgus with 1-year follow-up. The mean hallux valgus angle decreased from 36.2° preoperatively to 15.3° postoperatively. The intermetatarsal angle also improved significantly from 13.6° to 7.5°, and 87% of patients reported good to excellent results. Coetzee and colleagues[9] also recommend the Lapidus as the preferred procedure for salvage of failed hallux valgus surgery. They conducted a prospective cohort study of 26 feet with previously failed procedures. At 2 years, the mean AOFAS score had increased from 47.6 to 87.9 points. The mean intermetatarsal angle decreased from 18.0° to 8.6°.

Both the Keller arthroplasty and first metatarsophalangeal joint fusion may be preferred procedures for secondary hallux valgus operations. Kitaoka and colleagues[10] compared these procedures after failed hallux valgus surgery. Keller arthroplasty was performed on 11 feet, and first metatarsophalangeal joint fusion was performed on 9 feet. The mean age of each group was 63 years. In the resection arthroplasty group, the hallux valgus angle improved an average of 11°, whereas the intermetatarsal angle showed an improvement of 2°. In comparison, the arthrodesis subset showed a decrease in hallux valgus angle of 23° with an average 2° improvement in intermetatarsal angle. Results were good in 6 of the 11 feet in the arthroplasty group (54.5%) versus 6 of the 9 feet (67.0%) in the fusion group. The outcome of the joint-destructive procedure truly depends on proper patient selection. Younger, more active patients will have a more favorable result with an arthrodesis procedure. On the contrary, older and more sedentary patients may obtain adequate results with less healing and recovery time if a Keller arthroplasty is performed.

At University Foot & Ankle Institute, the most common finding for reoccurrence is either an undercorrected intermetatarsal angle or hypermobility of the first ray. In most cases, a Lapidus procedure with or without bone graft is undertaken rather than a reosteotomy. The authors have found that the Lapidus procedure allows proper alignment of the first ray in multiple planes and also allows for correction of length and possible hypermobility issues. Care should be taken when performing a second osteotomy on the first metatarsal because of an increased risk of nonunion, avascular necrosis, and scar formation. Finally, if a McBride-type bunionectomy was performed initially with no osteotomy, a Lapidus or proper osteotomy may be considered to correct the underlying problems.

MALUNION

One of the most common causes of failure is malunion. The most common type of malunion is caused by iatrogenic plantarflexion or dorsiflexion of the first metatarsal. This deformity may occur at surgery or may be a postoperative complication from early unendorsed weight-bearing by the patient. Most plantarflexion cases are iatrogenic and must be addressed at the time of surgery. Mild plantarflexion of the first ray is often desired to compensate for the mild shortening associated with first metatarsal osteotomies. However, if the fist metatarsal is too plantarflexed compared with its normal position, sesamoid pain and capsular inflammation about the first metatarsophalangeal joint may be noted. Care should be taken to check the position of the first ray before fixation on a lateral fluoroscopic image. If the osteotomy places the ray very plantar, the osteotomy should be dorsally displaced. If plantarflexion is noted after surgery, a cushioned shoe or an orthotic with a cutout under the first metatarsal may be helpful. If the region is still painful, a dorsiflexion osteotomy of the first ray may be necessary.

More common than plantarflexion of the first ray is elevation. An elevated first ray is commonly symptomatic and results in transfer lesions under the second metatarsal head, lateral column overload from the forefoot varus position, and possible midfoot arthritis of the lesser rays. Dorsiflexion problems may be iatrogenic or related to patient noncompliance. During surgery, the position of the first ray must be checked to ensure the metatarsal is not elevated. Well-designed osteotomies and rigid, stable internal fixation are essential in avoiding dorsiflexion of the first ray during the postoperative period. V-shaped osteotomies tend to be more stable and are therefore able to resist loading stress well compared with less-stable wedge osteotomies.[3] Care should be taken to avoid early weight-bearing, especially in patients in whom risk of dorsiflexion with increased plantar pressure is high. Should dorsal malunion of the first ray occur, an orthotic with a medial forefoot posting can help increase pressure under the first metatarsal region and improve pressure distribution. If this is not successful, plantarflexion of the first metatarsal either with osteotomy or with a Lapidus-type procedure, with or without bone grafting, can be helpful.

Hallux Varus

Hallux varus is another frequent problem related to hallux valgus correction. The main causes of hallux varus are iatrogenic and can occur with bunion correction, even in the best of surgical cases. One retrospective study found 4 resulting instances of iatrogenic hallux varus out of 270 Chevron bunionectomies performed, all of which required surgical intervention.[2] A common cause of varus deformity is overstacking of the medial eminence. This circumstance can be avoided by leaving the medial sesamoid groove intact. Overly aggressive closure of the intermetatarsal angle below zero can also cause hallux varus. The position of the first ray and distal osteotomy should be checked before final position fixation. If the alignment is not correct, adjustments at the time of surgery to the intermetatarsal angle should be made before final fixation. One of the most common causes of hallux varus is overtightening of the capsule medially. This condition results in a medial overhang of the tibial sesamoid, which can result in hallux varus. Finally, an aggressive lateral release with or without a fibular sesamoid removal results in poor tendon and ligament balance about the great toe joint, leading to varus formation. In all cases, proper intraoperative vigilance can help prevent a subsequent varus. Proper ray positioning, limited lateral release, and proper capsular balancing are essential surgical factors in avoiding hallux varus complications. Of interest with respect to different osteotomy options for hallux valgus correction is the possibility that some osteotomies have a higher risk of developing a varus than others. Although no research is available on the potential causes of hallux varus due to an opening wedge osteotomy, the authors believe that through lengthening the first metatarsal at an angle, the flexor tendon complex is put on stretch medially, resulting in an increased risk of hallux varus. Special attention should be given to the proper positioning of the first metatarsal in an opening wedge procedure to avoid overlengthening and possible risk of hallux varus.

Should a hallux varus complication occur, multiple options are available for correction. The most simple corrective action is strapping of the region. In some patients, strapping of the great toe to the lateral fifth metatarsal region is sufficient to relieve pain. Should surgery be necessary, a soft tissue release rarely works but can be attempted as a first-line option during surgery. Plovanich and colleagues[11] conducted a systematic review to assess the integrity of soft tissue reconstruction for flexible iatrogenic hallux varus repair. They found a 16.2% complication rate among all procedures. Transfer of the extensor hallucis longus tendon with fusion of the hallux interphalangeal joint was the only procedure to result in recurrence of the hallux varus with a rate of 4.4%. The other procedures performed included transfers of the abductor hallucis tendon, the first dorsal interosseous tendon, and the extensor hallucis brevis tendon. A tightrope procedure or internal brace technique for reefing of the lateral capsule and ligament structures can help reposition the ray. If the first intermetatarsal angle is dramatically overcorrected, a reverse medially shifting head osteotomy can realign the sesamoid complex and assist in hallux varus correction. One study found positive outcomes in varus correction with a reverse scarf osteotomy combined with opening wedge of the proximal phalanx after scarf/Akin osteotomies in a small subset of patients.[12] Others have suggested a reverse distal chevron osteotomy for cases in which the intermetatarsal angle has been overcorrected.[13] Often the authors will obtain patient consent for several procedures when hallux varus correction is planned. This practice allows each step to be systematically performed during surgery until great toe alignment is rectus. This procedure includes a soft tissue release, capsular release, ligament reefing, and possible metatarsal osteotomy. A fusion of the great toe joint is usually previously planned and not part of the systematic procedure. If the ray is rigidly positioned medially and/or arthritis of the first ray has occurred, a fusion of the first metatarsophalangeal joint can be the best option. Grimes and Coughlin[14] studied the results of first metatarsophalangeal joint fusion after failed surgical correction of hallux valgus and found satisfactory outcomes, including in patients who presented with iatrogenic hallux varus. Other investigators have also recommended fusion for failed hallux valgus surgery, because the influences around the first metatarsophalangeal joint may be unpredictable after an already unsuccessful procedure. First metatarsophalangeal joint arthrodesis assures permanent stability across the joint with little risk of subsequent deformity.[3]

Shortening

Iatrogenic shortening of the first metatarsal from osteotomy is yet another possible complication associated with hallux valgus surgery. The main causes of shortening are a poorly planned surgical procedure, a poorly performed metatarsal osteotomy, or possible shortening of the first metatarsal postoperatively because of poor bone quality or fixation failure.

Poor surgical planning most often results from performing the wrong procedure on an already short first metatarsal. If a short first metatarsal is present, a closing base wedge–type procedure or a Lapidus-type procedure with bone wedge cuts may result in excessive shortening. Potential alternatives include an opening base wedge osteotomy or a Lapidus with joint curettage with or without bone grafting. The use of the proper procedure based on the needs and requirements of each individual patient is essential for adequate outcome prediction.

Iatrogenic intraoperative shortening of the first metatarsal may also occur because of the osteotomy made. It is essential to consider that a head or base osteotomy should be made, at worst, perpendicular to the long axis of the first metatarsal to avoid shortening. A Kirschner wire (K-wire) can be used as an osteotomy guide and checked under fluoroscopic guidance before performing an osteotomy. In a minimally short first metatarsal, the osteotomy should be made to slightly lengthen the capital fragment relative to the long axis of the first metatarsal, which can help increase pressure on the first ray.

Shortening because of bone shift or fixation failure is also a common cause of hallux valgus complication. In an attempt to allow early weight-bearing, some cases may result in failure. The bone quality of each patient must be assessed at the time of surgery. If bone quality is deemed poor, a period of limited or non–weight-bearing can be helpful to avoid shortening of the first metatarsal from compression or bone failure. Furthermore, if fixation is deemed to be poor, a second point of fixation may be added, such as another screw, a plate, K-wire, or an absorbable pin. In the authors' practice, 2 screws are often placed in distal head osteotomies and 2 screws and a plate are placed on Lapidus bunionectomies to avoid fixation complications.

Should shortening occur, a lengthening scarf-type osteotomy or a bone-lengthening with bone graft may be attempted. Bevilacqua and colleagues[15] studied the amount of length obtained with a distraction scarf osteotomy in patients for whom previous bunion correction failed. They documented an increase in length of 7.08%, with a statistically significant increase between preoperative and postoperative measurements. They also described using the distraction scarf osteotomy in conjunction with a Lapidus procedure to maintain length of the metatarsal. This adjunct procedure prevented severe shortening in patients who were noted to have an already shortened first metatarsal preoperatively. If the main source of pain is transfer pressure on the lesser metatarsals, especially the second metatarsal, a shortening osteotomy of the lesser metatarsals may be a better option to compensate for the deranged length of the first metatarsal. Conservative options to help with first metatarsal shortening include stiff-soled rocker-style shoes, such as platforms, clogs, or wedges for women, which avoid the roll and push-off phases of gait and decrease forefoot overload. An orthotic with a metatarsal pad and a cutout under the second metatarsal with or without a Morton extension below the first metatarsal can be helpful to decrease pressure under the lesser metatarsals.

NONUNION

Nonunions are rare in hallux valgus surgery but can be a devastating problem to handle. Nonunions can be a result of either technical complications by the surgeon or issues related to the patient. Surgeon complication is often related to poor osteotomy or joint preparation and poor fixation. The osteotomy site must be prepared properly, including protection of the periosteum and joint capsule that supply nutrition to the bone. The actual osteotomy or joint resection should be performed with minimal thermal necrosis to avoid loss of vital cells necessary for bone healing. Finally, the area must be properly fixated to avoid movement and allow for bone integration and repair. Movement may cause scar tissue formation, which increases the chance of nonunion.

A second and less commonly considered cause of nonunion is patient-related issues, such as nutritional factors and/or poor compliance. These issues must be addressed before surgery to avoid postoperative issues. For example, if nutrition issues or potential bone quality and healing issues are considered a possibility, vitamin and bone density levels may need to be determined before surgery. Vitamins B and D are essential for proper healing. A low bone density level may result in poor bone healing and should be addressed with medication before surgery. Finally, patient compliance with weight-bearing status is critical to healing. Patients must be educated and instructed regarding the essential factors associated with non–weight-bearing and the potential for nonunion.

If the unfortunate scenario of a nonunion occurs, nutritional, bone density, and vitamin levels should be checked. Several bone density medications may be helpful in increasing bone healing. A bone scan can also help determine whether the nonunion is active or nonactive. A nonactive nonunion requires surgical care, because the region does not have good blood supply for healing. In these cases, removal of the nonunion, stable fixation, and possible bone grafting in an optimized patient can result in revision fusion. Hamilton and colleagues[16] conducted a multicenter retrospective study to evaluate the rate of union after revisional Lapidus for previously failed unions. Of the 17 feet receiving a bone-block Lapidus arthrodesis with autogenous bone grafting, 14 feet demonstrated successful union. Of particular interest, all 3 failed revisions were in patients who were active smokers. A bone stimulator may also be helpful to add to the mix of a nonunion with or without revision surgery.

AVASCULAR NECROSIS

Avascular necrosis is another rare cause of problems related to hallux valgus surgery. Often the problem has an unknown cause, and little is known regarding why it may occur in one person and not another. Several factors must be considered during surgery to avoid avascular necrosis risks. Limiting the amount of periosteal dissection and bone stripping is of primary concern. A thorough understanding of the location and proper protection of the vascular supply to the first ray is also important. Finally, proper internal fixation and stable bone constructs limit the risk of avascular necrosis. One cadaveric study showed that the vascular supply to the metatarsal was better preserved with a long dorsal arm osteotomy versus a Chevron osteotomy, and concluded that the risk for necrosis with the latter is greater.[17]

Should avascular necrosis occur, it is usually limited and can be reversed with the use of a bone stimulator. Non–weight-bearing may also help in early cases. If avascular changes progress, bone resection, bone grafting, and fusion may be necessary. If a large amount of resection is required to remove all devitalized bone, a bone block arthrodesis is most likely required to maintain length and avoid transfer metatarsalgia.

SUMMARY

Failure of hallux valgus surgery is an inevitable occasional outcome for all surgeons and is part of the potential risks of bunion surgery. Dealing with the complications is often laborious and complicated, and experience with revision surgery is essential for proper planning and adequate outcome.

To limit the risks associated with hallux valgus complications, proper planning is critical. Appropriate medical workup must be obtained, and the patient must have a solid understanding of the postoperative course. The surgeon must choose a suitable procedure for the associated hallux valgus deformity. The idea of one procedure being ideal for all patients must be abandoned. Hypermobility, ray length, toe position, and cartilage alignment/tracking must be assessed for proper procedure selection. The surgery must be performed with care to protect the vascular and nutritional supply to the surgical site. The first ray must be positioned properly and fixated with adequate stability. Soft tissue balancing also must be addressed before closure of the wounds. After surgery, the foot must be protected properly, through both the surgeon's instructions and the patient's protection of the region.

With proper planning, optimal surgical care, and patient protection, many of the issues associated with hallux valgus failure can be avoided. The hope is that the information provided in this article will serve as a template and starting point for patient care considerations related to hallux valgus surgery.

REFERENCES

1. Austin DW, Leventen ED. A new osteotomy for hallux valgus. Clin Orthop 1981; 157:25–30.
2. Lagaay PM, Hamilton GA, Ford LA, et al. Rates of revision surgery using Chevron-Austin osteotomies, Lapidus arthrodesis and closing base wedge osteotomies for correction of hallux valgus deformity. J Foot Ankle Surg 2008;47:267–72.
3. Belczyk R, Stapleton JJ, Grossman JP, et al. Complications and revisional hallux valgus surgery. Clin Podiatr Med Surg 2009;26:475–84.
4. Okuda R, Kinoshita M, Yasuda T, et al. The shape of the lateral edge of the first metatarsal head as a risk factor for recurrence of hallux valgus. J Bone Joint Surg 2007;89:2163–72.
5. Lyons MC, Terol C, Visser J, et al. Recurrent hallux valgus: treatment considerations. Podiatry Institute Update 2009;26:169–73.
6. Bock P, Lanz U, Kröner A, et al. The Scarf osteotomy: a salvage procedure for recurrent hallux valgus in selected cases. Clin Orthop Relat Res 2010;468: 2177–87.
7. Lim JB, Huntley JS. Revisional surgery for hallux valgus with serial osteotomies at two levels. ScientificWorldJournal 2011;11:657–61.

8. Ellington JK, Myerson MS, Coetzee JC, et al. The use of the Lapidus procedure for recurrent hallux valgus. Foot Ankle Int 2011;32:674–80.

9. Coetzee JC, Resig SG, Kuskowski M, et al. The Lapidus procedure as salvage after failed surgical treatment of hallux valgus: a prospective cohort study. J Bone Joint Surg Am 2003;85A:60–5.

10. Kitaoka HB, Patzer GL. Arthrodesis versus resection arthroplasty for failed hallux valgus operations. Clin Orthop Relat Res 1998;347:208–14.

11. Plovanich EJ, Donnenwerth MP, Abicht BP, et al. Failure after soft-tissue release with tendon transfer for flexible iatrogenic hallux varus: a systematic review. J Foot Ankle Surg 2012;51:195–7.

12. Kannegieter E, Kilmartin TE. The combined reverse scarf and opening wedge osteotomy of the proximal phalanx for the treatment of iatrogenic hallux varus. Foot (Edinb) 2011;21:88–91.

13. Lee KT, Park YU, Young KW, et al. Reverse distal chevron osteotomy to treat iatrogenic hallux varus after overcorrection of the intermetatarsal 1-2 angle: a technique tip. Foot Ankle Int 2011;32(1):89–91.

14. Grimes JS, Coughlin MJ. First metatarsophalangeal joint arthrodesis as a treatment for failed hallux valgus surgery. Foot Ankle Int 2006;27(11):887–93.

15. Bevilacqua NJ, Rogers LC, Wrobel JS, et al. Restoration and preservation of first metatarsal length using the distraction scarf osteotomy. J Foot Ankle Surg 2008; 47(2):96–102.

16. Hamilton GA, Mullins S, Schuberth JM, et al. Revision Lapidus arthrodesis: rate of union in 17 cases. J Foot Ankle Surg 2007;46(6):447–50.

17. Weinraub GM, Meberg R, Steinberg JS. Vascular perfusion of the long dorsal arm versus chevron osteotomy: a cadaveric injection study. J Foot Ankle Surg 2004; 43(4):221–4.

Contemporary Approaches and Advancements to the Lapidus Procedure

Bob Baravarian, DPM[a,b,]*, Rotem Ben-Ad, DPM[b]

KEYWORDS

- Bunionectomy • Lapidus • Weight-bearing Lapidus • Hypermobility • Pronation
- Bunion deformity

KEY POINTS

- The Lapidus bunionectomy is the ideal bunion surgery for correction of hallux valgus deformity at its source.
- There is a dramatic decrease in reoccurrence of hallux valgus deformity with the Lapidus procedure.
- Joint preparation, proper alignment, and rigid fixation are critical to outstanding outcomes with the Lapidus procedure.
- By using a rigid plate fixation, the Lapidus bunion procedure allows for early to immediate weight bearing with decreased downtime.

INTRODUCTION

The Lapidus procedure has long been considered one of the essential options for the correction of hallux valgus deformity. In a retrospective study of 47 feet, Catanzariti and colleagues[1] found no cases of hallux valgus recurrence. The average intermetatarsal angle reduced from 13.8 to 2.1. Only 3 nonunions resulted and 2 patients did go on to a hallux varus. For years, the procedure was considered the ideal option for large bunion deformities and hypermobility cases. The procedure continued to gain favor as the procedure of choice for hallux valgus correction overall because the underlying cause of the hallux valgus deformity was the laxity and hypermobility of the first ray at the metatarsocuneiform joint. By correcting the problem at the source of deformity without the use of osteotomy, the true cause of the bunion deformity is being addressed (**Fig. 1**). The main reasons for not performing the procedure were the

[a] Podiatric Foot and Ankle Surgery, Santa Monica UCLA Medical Center and Orthopedic Hospital, UCLA School of Medicine, Los Angeles, CA, USA; [b] University Foot and Ankle Institute, Los Angeles, CA, USA
* Corresponding author. Podiatric Foot and Ankle Surgery, Santa Monica UCLA Medical Center and Orthopedic Hospital, UCLA School of Medicine, Los Angeles, CA.
E-mail address: BBaravarian@mednet.ucla.edu

Clin Podiatr Med Surg 31 (2014) 299–308
http://dx.doi.org/10.1016/j.cpm.2014.01.001
0891-8422/14/$ – see front matter © 2014 Elsevier Inc. All rights reserved.

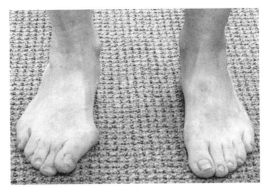

Fig. 1. Corrected bunion deformity with Lapidus procedure. Note corrected arch height and realignment and stabilization of midfoot after proper first ray realignment.

high rate of nonunion reported and the need for non–weight-bearing status by the patient. However, these issues are not able to be addressed with the more recent advancements in procedural technique. Current recovery periods after the Lapidus procedure seem comparable to other first ray procedures, such as a base wedge or head osteotomies.

WHY AVOID THE LAPIDUS PROCEDURE? MYTHS CONSIDERED

One of the main concerns about the Lapidus procedure was the high rates of nonunion. Early reports suggest rates as high as 25%.[2] More recent studies have demonstrated significantly lower nonunion rates. Patel and colleagues[3] found a nonunion rate of 5.3% in a review of 227 Lapidus procedures. The main sources of nonunion seem to be 3-fold. These are surgeon error-related problems, including poor internal fixation, poor joint preparation, and poor postoperative care. Other concerns that need to be considered are poor patient selection such as smokers, patients with poor nutritional status, and those with inadequate bone quality.

Another main concern, especially for the patient, is the prolonged period of non–weight bearing. The traditional recommendation has been complete non–weight bearing for a total of 6 to 8 weeks. This period is far longer than in head procedures but fairly equivalent to the amount of healing time required for base procedures. However, the authors present suggestions that have allowed them to keep patients ambulatory and limit the need for complete non–weight bearing.

A third reason often used by surgeons to avoid the Lapidus procedure as an option is that the incision usually is large and cosmetically may not be pleasing to the patient. We will also present our current treatment with a dual incision system, which has made our outcomes similar to any cosmetic-type head procedure with regard to incision healing (**Fig. 2**).

The final myth to be considered in the use of the Lapidus procedure is that limiting the movement of the first ray results in an abnormal stress on surrounding joints when compared with an osteotomy of the first ray; this is low on the scale of concerns noted by surgeons but has been addressed for completeness. In our 15-year follow-up history of patients undergoing Lapidus procedures, we have found no cases of surrounding arthritis from transfer of pressure. Furthermore, in dozens of patients with unilateral surgery performed, mainly because of previous surgery on the contralateral limb other than a Lapidus procedure, we have noted a dramatic difference in the rate of arthritis associated in surrounding joints on the non–Lapidus surgery foot. This condition may

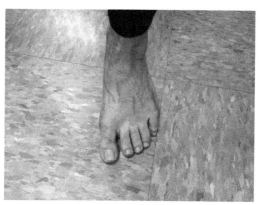

Fig. 2. Dual incision Lapidus procedure with cosmetic appearance of incision sites. Note dorsal midfoot incision and medial first metatarsal incision to break up appearance of one long dorsal scar.

be because the first ray is still mobile, or possibly hypermobile, at the first metatarso-cuneiform joint, which results in pressure transfer to the second ray, third ray, and naviculocuneiform joint.

PATIENT SELECTION

Patient selection is essential for proper and ideal outcomes after Lapidus procedure. What is presented is our personal selection process after 20 years of performing the procedure. Other surgeons may be either more liberal or slightly tougher on patient selection, but we have found our results consistent and solid with the use of the following patient selection criteria.

The patient must be able to understand the reasoning behind the procedure and the critical role they play in an adequate outcome. This criterion may seem simple but is the most essential part of the selection process. Patient weight, age, and bone quality can all be compensated for, but adequate understanding and compliance of the patient is critical and not under the physician's control. We have a deep and candid conversation with all patients, indicating the need not to smoke. Rates of nonunion with smokers have been dramatically higher than with nonsmokers. Patel and colleagues[4] performed a systematic review of the literature and found that 13 of the 17 studies examined determined smoking to have a deleterious effect on bone healing. We do not perform the procedure in a known smoker, especially if the smoking is daily and more than a casual case. We also avoid the Lapidus procedure in patients who are not clear on the amount of weight bearing allowed during the recovery period. Although we can allow patient full and immediate weight bearing on the foot after the Lapidus procedure, we want the option of deciding on that option based on the surgical procedure and bone quality. Therefore, patient compliance and the understanding of patient weight level are essential.

Patients also need to be nutritionally maintained, including bone quality and general nutritional factors. If a patient is considered questionable or if the surgeon believes there may be a nutritional issue with a patient, a vitamin level and possible bone density study may be performed. If bone quality is poor, the procedure is not performed. In most cases, the patient with minor to moderate bone density issues or vitamin insufficiency may be given vitamins D and B and may be referred to an osteoporosis specialist for bone density medications. We routinely have also begun using a vitamin pack for fusion cases, which includes vitamin B, vitamin D, and a stimulant for bone morphogenic protein, which seems to assist in bone healing and bone formation.

Considerations for juvenile bunions are stricter. We believe that hallux valgus in a young teen patient requires more dramatic and sustained correction. We have made a general policy to primarily attempt a Lapidus procedure in patients who have juvenile bunions. There may be limited one-time considerations for other procedures, but our patient selection of juvenile hallux valgus has resulted in far better short- and long-term outcomes with the use of the Lapidus procedure.

Another common source of debate related to the use of the Lapidus procedure is a patient with a short first ray. This condition has not been an issue in our hands. By using a curette technique instead of a joint resection technique and proper realignment of the ray in the sagittal, transverse, and coronal planes, a short ray can still be made to take proper weight in a virgin surgical case. In a case of iatrogenic shortening of the first ray from previous surgery, a Lapidus bunionectomy with the addition of a tricortical bone graft in the first metatarsocuneiform joint has allowed proper lengthening of the first ray and far better outcomes than an opening wedge procedure option.

Finally, many believe that the Lapidus procedure should be avoided in hallux valgus cases associated with arthritis of the first ray. Although we do not disagree with such cases on the far range of hallux limitus, we do believe that stage 2 to 3 hallux limitus cases associated with hallux valgus may still benefit from a Lapidus procedure with proper alignment of the first ray, decompression of the great toe joint, and removal of the abnormal spurring and arthritic changes in the great toe joint.

THE LAPIDUS SURGICAL PROCEDURE: THE UNIVERSITY FOOT AND ANKLE INSTITUTE TECHNIQUE

The patient is placed on the table in a supine position with a small bump under the ipsilateral hip to place the foot in a rectus position. Our preferred anesthesia is a popliteal fossa block with a long-acting local anesthetic and epinephrine unless contraindicated. Commonly, the patient receives a general anesthesia with the popliteal fossa block, as the block may take as long as 1 hour to take full effect, but in certain cases, a spinal anesthesia is used or appropriate time is taken for the block to take effect in which case mild or no sedation can be used. The reason for a popliteal fossa block is 24 to 48 hours of anesthesia for the patient after surgery, which has resulted in minimal need for pain medication and postoperative pain.

A tourniquet is placed at the calf level. The main reason for this positioning is that a thigh tourniquet is often painful for the patient and an ankle tourniquet does not allow proper hand positioning for placement of the proximal to distal screw fixation. Before elevation of the tourniquet, a stab incision is made on the lateral body of the calcaneus and a bone marrow aspiration is performed with a 30-mL syringe and a Jamshidi needle (**Fig. 3**). This bone aspirate is passed off the field, spun down and concentrated and mixed with a platelet-rich plasma taken from a vein puncture, and made into a gelatinous mix for later use. The Jamshidi needle is then used to harvest about 2 mL of bone graft from the heel to be used in the fusion site. The tourniquet is then inflated.

Our most common incision pattern is a dorsal incision over the first metatarsocuneiform joint combined with a medial incision at the metatarsophalangeal joint. We have not found it necessary to perform an incision in the first interspace and, rarely do we use an extensile dorsal incision. An extensile dorsal incision is used in revision cases with a previous incision or if a large fixation plate is necessary. The incision is taken to

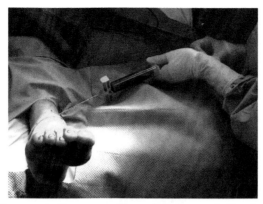

Fig. 3. Lateral heel bone aspiration process. The aspirate is passed off and spun down and combined with a platelet-rich plasma concentrate to make a gel that is placed in the fusion site.

the level of the tendon retinaculum protecting the neurovascular structures. The retinaculum is freed linearly and protected for later repair. The dorsal metatarsocuneiform joint is first opened. It is essential to protect the capsule for later repair, as it is one of the most important sources of nutrition and circulation to the joint. The joint is then distracted using a retractor of choice. Our preferred retractor is a Weinraub retractor, which allows k-wire pins to be placed in the first metatarsal and first cuneiform, which are then incorporated into holes in the distractor, which can then be spread open. The holes for the k-wires are made in the desired position for later screw placement (**Fig. 4**).

Following distraction of the joint, the cartilage is removed primarily with the use of an osteotome by hand. The osteotome is scraped against the cartilage, with limited to no removal of the subchondral bone. The plantar surface may need to be reached with a small straight rongeur or a small curette. It is okay to remove some minor subchondral bone on the edges or the plantar surfaces of the joint, but it is essential to leave the central portion intact, as this is the site the screws pass through the actual joint region. The subchondral bone is then fenestrated with a combination of 0.062 k-wire under lavage and a very small bone osteotome for shingling (**Fig. 5**). The region is lavaged and protected while the first metatarsophalangeal joint is exposed.

A medial incision is made in the first metatarsophalangeal joint. The joint is opened through a dorsal medial incision with a wedge taken out linearly for the redundant joint capsule. The size of the wedge taken out is based on the size and medial shift associated with the first ray. Minimal capsular dissection is performed to allow lateral release of the sesamoid collateral ligament. This procedure is done from an intra-articular approach. After the lateral sesamoid release, the lateral capsule is checked, and if tight, an intra-articular lateral release is performed through the lateral joint capsule. The toe is gently stressed medially to stretch the lateral capsule and ligaments. The medial eminence is then removed, taking care to leave the plantar medial sagittal groove intact; this is essential to avoid increased risk of hallux varus. If the toe is still found to pull laterally, the extensor hallucis brevis is transected at the proximal midfoot incision site. In certain cases in which preoperative examination shows rectus position of the toe and medial realignment of the toe, it may be possible to not open the great toe joint at all and only shift the metatarsal with a first metatarsocuneiform fusion. This method avoids scar formation and stiffening of the great toe joint, although this has been of little postoperative concern in our hands.

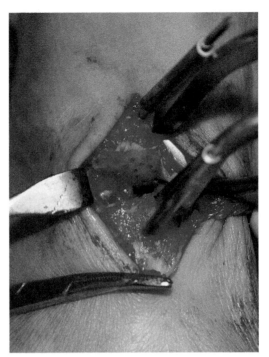

Fig. 4. Dorsal midfoot incision placement with distraction through the use of a laminar spreader with internal pin distractor. Note position of k-wires is also the desired position of screw placement.

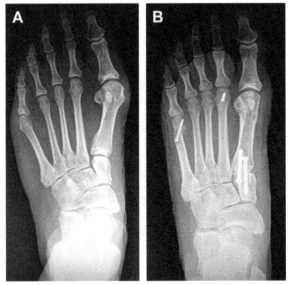

Fig. 5. (A) Preoperative radiograph of a hallux valgus deformity before screw fixation. (B) Initial fixation with crossed screw fixation. This procedure allows for excellent stabilization but does not allow for weight bearing.

After proper release of the great toe joint, the gelled stem cell/platelet-rich plasma material is placed in the first metatarsocuneiform joint and the metatarsal is positioned to as close to a zero intermetatarsal angle as possible. The bone graft from the heel is used to fill any small gaps that may have been produced, and fixation is undertaken.

Optimal internal fixation of the fusion site is essential for union rate and weight-bearing potential in the Lapidus procedure. Our initial fixation was crossed screw fixation, with the proximal-to-distal screw grabbing the metatarsal base (**Fig. 6**). With this technique, we did not allow weight bearing for 6 weeks or until adequate fusion seemed to be taking place. With the addition of the stem cell concentrate, we have seen early fusion on patients at 4 weeks, which began to speed up weight bearing to 4 weeks. However, we believe early weight bearing was essential to make the Lapidus procedure mainstream and available for all patients. We began to experiment with different plate fixation options. We have currently begun to use 2 plate options that are selected according to patient size, bone quality, and need for immediacy of weight bearing. Both plates offer a combination of locking and nonlocking options. The 2 plates differ in construct according to size and thickness. The more common plate system used is 1.4 mm in thickness, which is low profile. Five plate options are available in the Stryker 1.4 mm set, which include plates different in shape and length (**Fig. 7**). This one is essentially our primary set. In rare cases, we prefer a thicker and stronger plate, which is 1.6 to 1.8 mm in thickness at differing plate sites. This system by Orthofix (Lewisville, TX) is an excellent anatomic plate but far thicker. What is best about the Orthofix plate is that it may offer greater stability in a large patient with need for early weight bearing, and that is its primary use in Dr Baravarian practice.

The overall construct for fixation is done through crossing screws for primary compression followed by a dorsal medial plate fixation. The plate is positioned on the medial aspect to allow screws to run into the middle cuneiform and second metatarsal if need be.

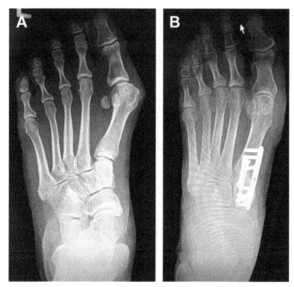

Fig. 6. (*A*) Preoperative radiograph of a hallux valgus deformity before thin plate and screw fixation. (*B*) Fixation of Lapidus bunionectomy with crossed screw compression and medial thin plate fixation.

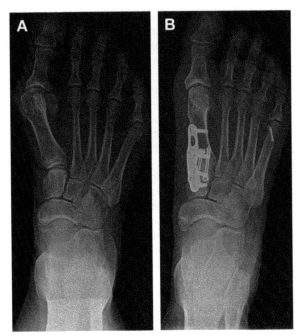

Fig. 7. (*A*) Preoperative radiograph of a hallux valgus deformity before thick plate and screw fixation. (*B*) Fixation of Lapidus bunionectomy with crossed screw compression and medial thin plate fixation. This method is used in heavyset patient or if added stability and immediate weight bearing is necessary.

After fixation, the remaining bone marrow aspirate concentrate is injected into the nooks about the fusion site and allowed to gel. Closure of the capsules is performed using the surgeon's choice of suture. Care is taken to close the first metatarsal-phalangeal joint capsule at a slight bias to medially shift the great toe and allow repositioning of the sesamoid complex.

The initial dressing is placed, followed by a fiberglass below the knee cast. The patient is seen 5 days postsurgery for an initial wound check and for a new cast to be placed.

TO WEIGHT BEAR OR NOT TO WEIGHT BEAR?

The concept of weight bearing after fusion surgery has advanced dramatically in the past 10 years. Surgeries that used to require prolonged periods of non–weight bearing are now performed with a dramatic decrease in the non–weight-bearing period, which truly began with spinal fusion, which did not lend well to non–weight-bearing periods. Subsequent techniques for fixation of the spine were adjusted to lower extremity surgery. During the past 5 years, foot and ankle weight bearing has become a concept of increased interest. Many cases are now weight bearing, which used to require prolonged non–weight bearing. These include Achilles repairs, calcaneal spur removal, hammer toe fusion procedures, plantar plate repairs, first metatarsophalangeal fusions, and now first ray hallux valgus procedures. Many base wedge procedures are now adjusted to allow early weight bearing. However, few articles about weight bearing of the Lapidus exist. Blitz and colleagues[5] performed a multicenter retrospective analysis of 80 feet in 76 patients who underwent a Lapidus procedure. Patients were allowed to begin protective weight bearing at 2 weeks. Mean time to complete union was 44.5 days, and no cases of nonunion were reported. No revision surgeries were necessary. All procedures were performed with either 2 or 3 crossed screws without any plate fixation. Sorensen and colleagues[6] demonstrated that locking plate fixation also allowed for early weight bearing at 2 weeks with fusion rates of 100%. One study even demonstrated 100% union in 27 Lapidus procedures after allowing patient to weight bearing immediately in a wedge shoe.[7]

Our weight bearing habits have changed with an increased understanding of the healing process associated with the Lapidus procedure. Although screw fixation and weight bearing may be possible, we do not think cannulated screws allow adequate support for early weight bearing. However, with the additional bone marrow aspirate, we have seen fusions at as early at 4 weeks, which has allowed early weight bearing for some patients with simple crossed cannulated screw fixation.

Our preferred fixation with crossed cannulated screws and a locking plate system has allowed us to begin early weight bearing, which was first started with partial weight at 4 weeks postsurgery. We then progressed to partial weight of about 20% at 2 weeks and gradually increased to 100% at 4 weeks. During the course of 2 years, this process was checked and no nonunions were seen. We have now progressed partial weight at 5 days postsurgery with increase to full weight at between 2 and 3 weeks postsurgery at which time sutures are removed. A removable boot is then fitted to allow range of motion exercises, physical therapy, and washing of the region. Boot removal and progression to a stiff shoe is usually at about 5 weeks. To date, we have still not seen a single nonunion in 3 years using this current fixation, marrow aspirate, and weight-bearing progression system.

SUMMARY

The Lapidus procedure is truly the ideal hallux valgus correction option. Return of the hallux valgus deformity is far lower with a Lapidus procedure than with other bunion surgeries, and that procedure allows for anatomic correction of the underlying deformity and joint laxity issues. The Lapidus procedure also stabilizes the medial column of the foot and decreases abnormal stress and potential arthritis of the midfoot and other metatarsal cuneiform joints. The Lapidus procedure also can help with reduction of lateral column compression symptoms associated with first ray elevatus.

The commonly associated complications of the Lapidus procedure have included nonunion, shortening of the first ray, poor cosmetic scar formation on the dorsum of the foot, and need for prolonged non–weight bearing. During the past 5 years, University Foot and Ankle Institute has undertaken a new and contemporary approach to dealing with the aforementioned associated complications to make the Lapidus procedure more attainable to all patients requiring hallux valgus correction. To that end, we have taken the surgery apart and broken it down and improved the portions to create a better overall outcome. To avoid shortening of the ray, the only cartilage is removed and the subchondral bone is left intact and fenestrated. By not using a saw to make bone cuts, we have avoided the shortening issues. To avoid a long and possibly noncosmetic scar on the dorsum of the foot, we make a dorsal cuneiform region incision and a medial metatarsophalangeal incision. The medial incision heals well, and the cuneiform incision also heals with minimal scarring, and because both scars are smaller than one long dorsal scar, the incisions are "broken apart" and less visible. The nonunion and non–weight-bearing issues are dealt with in the same manner. We have augmented the fusion with a small amount of calcaneal bone graft and a bone marrow/platelet-rich plasma concentrate cocktail, which is placed in the fusion site. Fixation is achieved with a construct of crossing screws at the fusion site and a dorsal medial locking plate fixation system. This system has allowed us to begin partial weight bearing at 5 days and full weight bearing at 2 to 3 weeks, with return to stiff shoe gear at about 5 weeks. This result is comparable to other osteotomy-type bunion surgeries, including head osteotomies. To date, this construct has not resulted in a single nonunion, and we believe immediate weight bearing postsurgery may be possible in certain patient groups who do not have other complicating factors such as poor bone quality, high body mass index, or poor coordination.

With time and increased research, foot and ankle surgery is progressing to a level never thought possible. Improved fixation and an improved knowledge of soft tissue and bone healing have allowed for dramatic advancements in hallux valgus correction and made the Lapidus procedure our preferred surgery.

REFERENCES

1. Catanzariti AR, Mendicino RW, Lee MS, et al. The modified Lapidus arthrodesis: a retrospective analysis. J Foot Ankle Surg 1999;38(5):322–32.
2. Blitz NM. The versatility of the Lapidus arthrodesis. Clin Podiatr Med Surg 2009; 26:427–41.
3. Patel S, Ford LA, Etcheverry J, et al. Modified Lapidus arthrodesis: rate of nonunion in 227 cases. J Foot Ankle Surg 2004;43(1):37–42.
4. Patel RA, Wilson RF, Patel PA, et al. The effect of smoking on bone healing: a systematic review. Bone Joint Res 2013;2(6):102–11.
5. Blitz NM, Lee T, Williams K, et al. Early weight bearing after modified Lapidus arthrodesis: a multicenter review of 80 cases. J Foot Ankle Surg 2010;49(4): 357–62.
6. Sorensen MD, Hyer CF, Berlet GC. Results of Lapidus arthrodesis and locked plating with early weight bearing. Foot Ankle Spec 2009;2(5):227–33.
7. Kazzaz S, Singh D. Postoperative cast necessity after Lapidus arthrodesis. Foot Ankle Int 2009;30(8):746–51.

Physical Therapy Post–Hallux Abducto Valgus Correction

Suzanne T. Hawson, PT, MPT, OCS

KEYWORDS

- Physical therapy • Bunion • Hallux abducto valgus • Postoperative rehabilitation
- Bunionectomy

KEY POINTS

- Corrective surgery for hallux valgus is an option when conservative measures fail.
- Hallux valgus has biomechanical implications that affect the entire functional chain, and these issues may not correct themselves postoperatively.
- A comprehensive physical therapy evaluation for postoperative hallux valgus correction is needed to identify problems and diagnose movement dysfunction that may lead to disability and affect how an individual interacts with the environment.
- A multifaceted physical therapy program addresses impairments and functional limitations to help restore normal function centered on patient-specific goals.

INTRODUCTION

Hallux valgus is a fairly common occurrence. In a cross-sectional study performed in 2010, Nix and colleagues[1] found that the prevalence of hallux valgus was 23.0% in adults aged 18 to 65 years and 35.7% in adults older than 65 years. Hallux valgus is more prevalent in women and elderly (>65 years of age) individuals.[1]

Many treatments can be considered for hallux valgus. Conservative measures, such as orthotics, physical therapy, footwear modifications, and injections, have been documented as ways to treat this condition, and although conservative measures do not correct the deformity itself, they can help reduce pain and improve function.[2]

However, when conservative measures do not yield the desired result and symptoms such as pain persist in not only the big toe but also the other digits, surgical correction is often considered.[2] Surgical osteotomy for hallux valgus was shown to be effective for treating painful hallux valgus, whereas orthoses provided only short-term relief.[3] Procedures may vary from osteotomy of the first metatarsal to addressing involvement at the tarsometatarsal joint and/or the proximal phalanx.[2]

The author has nothing to disclose.
Department of Physical Therapy, University Foot and Ankle Institute, 26357 McBean Parkway, Suite 250, Valencia, CA 91355, USA
E-mail address: suzanne@footankleinstitute.com

Clin Podiatr Med Surg 31 (2014) 309–322
http://dx.doi.org/10.1016/j.cpm.2014.01.002
0891-8422/14/$ – see front matter © 2014 Elsevier Inc. All rights reserved.

Several types of surgical procedures are used in treating hallux valgus, but describing them in detail is beyond the scope of this article. In general, mild deformities would be less involved than severe deformities (Wulker[2]), and additional procedures may be needed to address other issues, such as a Lapidus procedure for tarsometatarsal joint instability.[4] Surgery addresses the different joints that constitute the first ray and corrects the deformity for optimal joint function, and may include addressing issues in the first tarsometatarsal, metatarsophalangeal, and the proximal interphalangeal (PIP) joints. In general, proper surgical treatment results in good outcomes in 85% of patients.[2] However, the severity and chronicity of the hallux valgus deformity before surgery could also potentially affect a patient's prognosis. These patients may continue to have symptoms leading to impaired body functions, limited function from disuse, and altered biomechanical function, which might limit or delay expected outcomes.

Currently, the American Podiatry Medical Association (APMA) Web site mentions physical therapy as a treatment for hallux valgus specifically to "provide relief of the inflammation and bunion pain" and that postsurgical pain can be managed with medications, without mention of physical therapy.[5] The American Academy of Orthopedic Surgeons (AAOS) Web site mentions physical therapy as part of postoperative care after bunion surgery to help with exercises.[6] Consequently, physical therapy may be underused in postoperative hallux valgus correction. This article highlights the usefulness of physical therapy to help regain function and optimize outcomes for patients who undergo hallux valgus surgery.

Physical therapists are qualified medical professionals who diagnose and manage movement dysfunction and enhance physical and functional abilities.[7] In 2008, the World Health Organization established the International Classification of Functioning. This system focuses on human function, providing a framework for how people with particular health conditions function in their daily lives. Alterations in body function, rather than a particular diagnosis, can affect how individuals can perform normal tasks and their interaction with the environment. Physical therapists consider all of these factors and address them when planning a treatment plan and providing care.[8]

Postoperative physical therapy is indicated for patients who have undergone hallux valgus correction who have altered body functions and disability resulting from surgery, and to address symptoms and biomechanical issues that are associated with hallux valgus. Postoperatively, patients may present with pain, edema, impaired range of motion, impaired muscle strength and function, joint dysfunction in the foot and ankle complex, possible nerve dysfunction, altered balance, integumentary changes, and gait disturbance. Functional ability and patient expectations may fall short without proper intervention after hallux valgus correction. Although some of these issues are sequelae of surgery, studies have shown that strength and proper foot function associated with hallux valgus may not correct themselves without proper treatment, even after surgical correction,[9–11] and that physical therapy is helpful to improve weight-bearing forces on the hallux and first ray after hallux valgus surgery.[12]

COMPREHENSIVE EXAMINATION AND TREATMENT OF POSTSURGICAL HALLUX VALGUS

Physical therapists conduct an initial examination in which patient history, a systems review, and tests and measures are completed to evaluate and establish a plan of care that outlines diagnosis, goals, interventions, and prognosis. Gathering subjective information from patients regarding their history helps physical therapists determine which tests and measures should be completed, and provides information on functional limitations and patients' goals and expected outcome, which must be considered when establishing the plan of care.[7]

A systems review quickly determines the status of body systems, such as the integumentary system, gross symmetry of the musculoskeletal system, neuromuscular system, cardiovascular system, and communication ability, if indicated.[7] For instance, screening for possible deep vein thrombosis should be completed especially when the patient complains of calf pain and tenderness. A prospective study by Solis and Saxby[13] showed that 7 of 201 patients who had foot and ankle surgery had deep vein thrombosis and that risk factors included immobilization, hindfoot surgery, tourniquet time, and advancing age.

Infection must also be ruled out as part of the systems review. Low-grade fever and redness, warmth, abnormal swelling, and induration of the incision at the surgical site may indicate the presence of an infection. If infection is suspected, the surgeon or treating physician should be notified. Skin integrity should be noted, such as the presence of wound dehiscence; otherwise, an assessment of scar mobility should be completed.

According to the APTA Guide to Physical Therapy Practice, tests and measures help identify and characterize signs and symptoms of pathology/pathophysiology, impairments, functional limitations, and disabilities.[7] Physical therapists take the information gathered from the examination to evaluate dysfunction and prognosis, establish a movement diagnosis, and establish a plan of care that includes treatment interventions and goals. Interventions are designed to address specific impairments and functional limitations to meet outlined rehabilitation goals.

RESTORING NORMAL JOINT FUNCTION AFTER HALLUX VALGUS CORRECTION

Symptoms such as pain, impaired joint mobility, difficulty wearing shoes, altered gait, deformity, and reduced function, unresolved using conservative measures, typically lead to surgical correction.[2,14] Although surgical correction of hallux valgus deformity reduces the bony deformity and returns the proper bony alignment to the first ray, other symptoms may persist postoperatively. Given enough time and palliative care, these symptoms may resolve on their own. However, there is indication that dysfunction remains after hallux valgus surgery that does not necessarily resolve.[9–11] Physical therapy has been shown to help improve function after hallux valgus surgery,[15] and individuals with pain, loss of motion, and weakness improved with treatment such as mobilization, strengthening, and gait training.[16]

Postoperative pain may be limited to the foot and ankle region; however, it may extend up along the kinetic chain from gait deviations or from prolonged immobilization postoperatively. Pain may be incisional or neurogenic, arise from inflammation of the joint capsule and/or surrounding soft tissue structures, or be related to limited mobility. Obtaining information regarding the quality, frequency, intensity, and description of pain helps therapists determine the cause of the pain and address it properly. Scales or tests and measures of pain and disability, such as the Foot Function Index, have been shown to be valid and reliable tools for determining foot health.[17] Addressing the source of pain, such as limited range of motion at the metatarsophalangeal joint causing discomfort during terminal stance and preswing phases of gait, can help reduce symptoms.

Impaired range of motion is one of the most common reasons for referral to physical therapy postoperatively. Range of motion of the PIP and metatarsophalangeal joint of the hallux may be limited by pain, edema, connective tissue restrictions in the joint capsule, soft tissue restrictions such as scarring, lack of muscle flexibility, and impaired tendon gliding. Kernozek and Sterriker[10] report that after Chevron-Akin osteotomy, patients had decreased dorsiflexion range of motion at the hallux metatarsophalangeal joint, which would affect normal gait pattern and can contribute to complaints of pain.

Performing range of motion activities in the hallux metatarsophalangeal and PIP joints can be difficult if pain is severe. This discomfort can cause joint and muscle guarding and compensatory gait techniques to avoid movement in the painful area. Maitland grades I and II joint mobilization techniques to oscillate the metatarsophalangeal and PIP joints can reduce pain and muscle guarding. Other techniques, such as application of transcutaneous electrical nerve stimulation (TENS), can be beneficial to manage pain. Brief intense TENS can be used to help anesthetize the hallux to allow mobilization of a painful joint and reduce guarding from pain,[18] enabling joint mobilization. Other modalities, such as electrical stimulation, ultrasound, and cryotherapy, can also reduce muscle guarding and release trigger points,[18] and low-level laser therapy has been shown to reduce joint pain in patients.[19]

Sometimes, patients present with a complaint of sensitivity and altered sensation in the foot and ankle area postoperatively. Nerve dysfunction at the common superficial peroneal nerve and sural nerve may result from surgery. A direct mechanical lesion or tourniquet-related ischemia and conduction-block that affect normal nerve function are potential risks of surgery.[20] The altered sensation may be described as pain, numbness or tingling, impaired sensation to light touch, or sensitivity to objects touching the affected areas, and may potentially affect the person's footwear choices. Pain of this nature can be addressed with physical modalities, manual therapy, and desensitization techniques.[7]

Incisional scarring can also contribute to pain in the hallux and may limit normal joint function. One study reported that 31% of patients reported nerve-type issues with their scar after hallux valgus surgery, but many of these issues resolved with time and without surgical intervention.[21] The lack of scar mobility may inhibit range of motion at the metatarsophalangeal and interphalangeal joints, limiting functional movement needed for gait.

Improved scar appearance has been observed with the use of silicone, pressure therapy, exercise,[22] and a combination of silicone gel and vitamin C,[23] and silicone gel sheets have been found to reduce hypertrophic and keloid scarring.[24] Low-level light therapy has been shown to help accelerate wound healing[25] and can reduce keloids.[26] Ultrasound is indicated for reducing scar formation when used in a pulsed setting.[18] Iodine iontophoresis, a process through which medication is administered with the use of electrical stimulation to deliver a chemical, has been shown to reduce scars.[27] In addition, manual therapy techniques to mobilize adhesions may be applied by the physical therapist, and patients should be educated on the proper technique and complete this activity as part of an independent home program.

Persistent swelling postoperatively can affect range of motion and is another common complaint of patients after undergoing surgery for hallux valgus. Anthropometric measurements of the foot, ankle, and calf using a tape measure or volumometer quantify the amount of swelling between the operative and nonoperative limb. Because footwear is a primary concern for patients with hallux valgus,[1,28] it will continue to be an issue postoperatively if edema, pain, and lack of joint mobility continue to limit footwear choices. Early in rehabilitation, a stiffer-soled shoe that limits movement in the forefoot and that can accommodate swelling of the foot and ankle areas can help to reduce painful weight-bearing dorsiflexion after hallux valgus correction.

Manual therapy techniques such as edema massage and lymph drainage can be used to address edema. Application of electrical stimulation, ultrasound, cryotherapy, iontophoresis, and taping may also reduce inflammation. The Kinesio Taping technique used for edema, together with lymphatic massage, has been shown to significantly reduce postoperative edema, and reduces it faster than lymphatic draining alone.[29] **Fig. 1** illustrates the application of Kinesio Tape for edema. The use of compression garments and range of motion exercises[30] have also been shown to reduce edema.

Reducing the appearance of the bunion deformity is the primary goal of hallux valgus surgery, and is achieved through reducing the lateral deviation of the hallux toward the second toe and improving alignment of the metatarsal. The bony deformity is addressed with surgery; however, with prolonged history of hallux valgus, the length of connective tissue in surrounding structures may have also undergone permanent deformation or creep[31] that can potentially make rehabilitation more involved. With hallux valgus, the medial ligaments are stretched with shortening of lateral structures, which disrupts normal hallux metatarsophalangeal joint function.[32] Soft tissues along the lateral side of the first metatarsophalangeal joint, specifically the adductor hallucis muscle attachment, are typically released during surgery. Partial tenotomy of the adductor hallucis and flexor hallucis brevis muscles with release of the lateral sesamoid ligament has been shown to reduce hallux valgus deformity.[33] However, postoperative immobilization may result in scarring, leading to hypomobility of these structures. This technique is also associated with a potential risk of deviation of the hallux toward the second toe, even after surgical correction.

In addition, muscle imbalance exists in patients with hallux valgus before surgery. Ultrasonic studies have also indicated that the abductor hallucis undergoes morphologic changes during the development of hallux valgus, which are associated with reduced strength of the abductor hallucis secondary to disuse.[34] The abductor

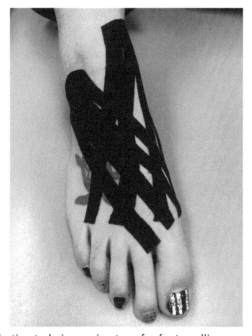

Fig. 1. Edema application technique using tape for foot swelling.

hallucis is found to be weaker for patients with a larger hallux valgus angle,[35] and the abductor hallucis has been found to be weaker than the adductor hallucis.[36] This muscle imbalance is not automatically corrected by surgery and will require proper strengthening exercises to prevent drifting of the hallux toward the second toe. Manual techniques for stretching soft tissues and mobilizations to the joint capsule and intermetatarsal joints can help reduce soft tissue restrictions. Taping and other equipment, such as toe spacers or bunion splints, can also be used postoperatively to help improve toe alignment (**Fig. 2**).

Restoring proper function of the sesamoids improves forefoot mechanics needed for proper gait. Preoperatively, hallux valgus affects the resting position of the sesamoids as it is pushed into the medial capsular wall of the joint,[37] causing erosion of cartilage and damaging the subchondral bone on the metatarsal head.[37] The sesamoids are laterally displaced by hallux valgus, and when the deformity is severe, the lateral sesamoid dislocates lateral to the first metatarsal head and the medial sesamoid ends up in the groove that originally corresponded to the lateral sesamoid.[38] Studies have shown that hallux valgus surgery likely relocates the first metatarsal on top of the sesamoids,[39,40] but clinically, impaired sesamoid mobility and painful sesamoids are noted postoperative in patients who have undergone hallux valgus correction.

A comprehensive intervention program for limited hallux range of motion should include great toe mobilization, toe flexor strengthening, and sesamoid bones mobilization.[41] Good sesamoid mobility contributes to improved gait pattern in patients with hallux limitus.[16] Therefore, ensuring proper sesamoid function postoperatively is important after hallux valgus correction. Techniques such as transverse friction

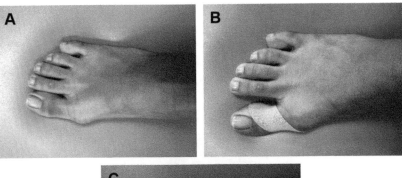

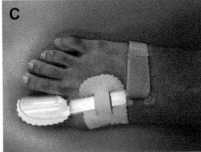

Fig. 2. (*A*) Resting position for hallux valgus. Note deviation of hallux toward second toe. (*B*) Use of 1-inch tape to reduce deviation. (*C*) Use of PediFix bunion splint to reduce deviation of the hallux.

massage to the flexor hallucis longus, soft tissue work to intrinsic foot muscles, sesamoid mobilizations and exercises are discrete entities that can help improve sesamoid mobility, resulting in improved forefoot function.

Limited joint capsular mobility as a result of immobilization may contribute to impaired range of motion at the hallux metatarsophalangeal and PIP joints. Hypomobility of the joint capsule would limit plantarflexion and dorsiflexion of the metatarsophalangeal joint, requiring joint mobilization techniques. Specifically, grade III/IV joint mobilizations are used to bring connective tissue past its yield zone and into the plastic phase of elongation to make a permanent change in the tissue length.[31] In addition, dynamic splinting has been shown to be effective in reducing postoperative contracture for hallux limitus, involving the use of a dynamic splint for the first metatarsophalangeal joint for 60 minutes 3 times a day to help regain hallux metatarsophalangeal joint dorsiflexion.[42] The use of passive motion devices after the Austin procedure improves rehabilitation time and enables quicker return to wearing shoes compared with physical therapy alone.[43]

A primary goal in reducing pain and swelling and regaining normal joint function is to have the appropriate range of motion for normal gait. Normal gait requires $55°$ to $60°$ of hallux metatarsophalangeal degree of freedom in the sagittal plane.[44,45] Limited dorsiflexion of the hallux metatarsophalangeal joint would lead to a diminished toe rocker required for normal gait propulsion. The toe rocker allows for smooth forward progression of the trailing stance limb. Patients who undergo the Lapidus procedure, who are immobilized for a longer period to ensure fusion of the first metatarsocuneiform joint, may present with more joint hypomobility and atrophy in the lower leg from the immobilization period. The tarsometatarsal, intermetatarsal, talocrural, and subtalar joints should also be assessed, because normal functioning of these joints contributes to proper gait. In patients who undergo a Lapidus procedure to stabilize the first metatarsocuneiform (tarsometatarsal joint), this joint should not be mobilized.

Restoring normal gait pattern after hallux valgus correction not only relies on having normal range of motion in multiple joints but also requires strength and proper muscle timing. Normal toe-off requires normal strength of the hallux plantarflexors (flexor hallucis longus and flexor hallucis brevis).[44] Hallux plantarflexion strength has been documented to decrease in patients with hallux valgus. Impaired plantar loading of the hallux and increased load on the lateral surface of the foot have been found preoperatively and postoperatively in patients who undergo hallux valgus correction.[9,10] Postoperative physical therapy has been shown to be associated with decreased load-bearing on the hallux[11] and improved weight-bearing on the hallux and the first ray.[12] Weakness of the flexor hallucis longus and flexor digitorum longus decreases hallux contact force and increased forces under the lateral metatarsal heads.[46]

Assessing overall foot and ankle muscle function postoperatively will likely reveal continued strength issues. Strength of other extrinsic musculature such as the peroneus longus should be assessed, because the peroneus longus helps pronate the first ray to contact the ground during gait.[44] According to Jacob[47], the flexor hallucis longus and brevis tendons and the peroneus longus muscle exert a resultant force on the first metatarsal head amounting to 119% of body weight during loading phase of gait. Gastrocnemius and soleus function should be tested, because these muscles play a large role in decelerating the limb during weight acceptance[45]; however, the completion of standardized testing of the gastrocnemius and soleus may be limited by recent surgery, because assessment requires unilateral heel rises.[48] Heel rise requires $58°$ of hallux metatarsophalangeal joint dorsiflexion,[49] and if range of motion is limited, then the test cannot be completed in a valid manner.

The overall function of the lower extremity, from the foot to the pelvic girdle, can be altered because of forces acting on the foot.[50] Patients with a long history of hallux valgus may potentially have issues proximally along the kinetic chain, including the knee, hip, and pelvis. Functional tests, such as squatting, climbing, reaching, and other activities directly related to a patient's specific concern, are administered by physical therapists. These tests provide useful information related to weight-bearing activities and can give the therapist information on strength and muscle timing/control issues along the kinetic chain that relate to functional activities. Hip exercises to improve mechanics and balance exercises are needed, because increased medial/lateral postural sway has been found in people with hallux abducto valgus.[35] Some basic exercises that are helpful for regaining strength after hallux valgus correction are shown in **Figs. 3–5**.

Proper leg muscle function helps improve balance postoperatively. Impaired balance as a result of pain, edema, impaired muscle function, impaired joint proprioceptive awareness, and impaired timing and coordination may affect static and dynamic balance. Impaired balance is a risk factor for falling. Foot pain impairs balance and functional mobility in older people,[51] which may increase risk of falling.

Foremost, physical therapists address patients' ability to complete normal functional activities of daily living and how patients interact with their environment. The person's ability to wear particular shoes comfortably, complete activities such as walking to/from different rooms within their home, climb up and down stairs, and resume normal exercise activities are all functions that may be affected by hallux valgus surgery. Several functional questionnaires are available for assessing function when addressing foot and ankle conditions, such as the American Orthopaedic Foot & Ankle Society scales, Visual Analog Scale, Short Form-36 Health Survey, and the Foot Function Index.[17,52] The Foot and Ankle Ability Measure, Foot Function Index, Foot Health Status Questionnaire, and Lower Extremity Function Scale are considered to have content validity, construct validity, reliability, and responsiveness.[53]

Several factors should be considered when dealing with this specific population. For instance, the complexity of the surgical procedure, existing biomechanical issues that may have predisposed the patient to hallux valgus deformity, and patient expectations regarding outcomes can all affect the rate of success of surgery. Other factors,

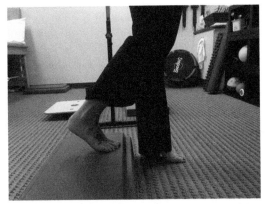

Fig. 3. Weight-bearing dorsiflexion over the metatarsophalangeal joints. Patients are instructed to apply plantar pressure over the hallux and avoid favoring lesser metatarsals.

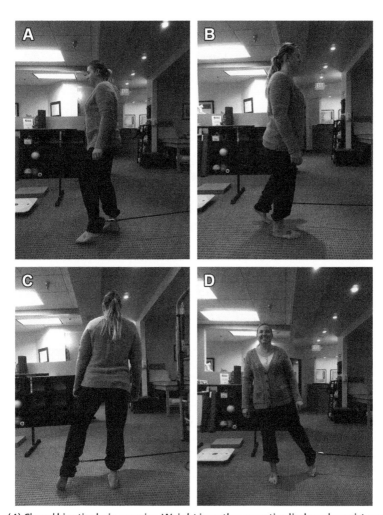

Fig. 4. (A) Closed kinetic chain exercise. Weight is on the operative limb and a resistance band is applied to the contralateral limb. The patient is instructed to balance on the operative limb while pressing down on the hallux as the contralateral limb is moved in into flexion. (B) Closed kinetic chain exercise. Weight is on the operative limb and a resistance band is applied to the contralateral limb. The patient is instructed to balance on the operative limb while pressing down on the hallux as the contralateral limb is moved in into extension. (C) Closed kinetic chain exercise. Weight is on the operative limb and a resistance band is applied to the contralateral limb. The patient is instructed to balance on the operative limb while pressing down on the hallux as the contralateral limb is moved in into abduction. (D) Closed kinetic chain exercise. Weight is on the operative limb and a resistance band is applied to the contralateral limb. The patient is instructed to balance on the operative limb while pressing down on the hallux as the contralateral limb is moved in into adduction.

such as delayed union or nonunion, are also of concern. A systematic literature review found a nonunion rate of 5.4% and that 8.5% of patients required hardware removal.[54] Biomechanical issues associated with hallux valgus are well documented.[2,4,55–59] Altered foot mechanics such as abnormal pronation[4,55,56] and calcaneal eversion[58]

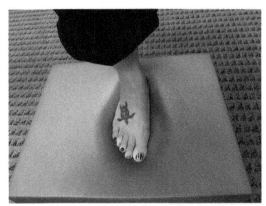

Fig. 5. Single-limb balance activity on a stability mat to challenge dynamic function of lower extremity muscles.

may not have been addressed during surgery for hallux valgus. If not addressed, then the use of orthoses postoperatively to address rearfoot motion and improve forefoot loading[2,35] would be an important part of the continuum of care to optimize lower extremity mechanics.

A comprehensive and patient-specific physical therapy treatment program is beneficial in maximizing outcomes of hallux valgus correction and improving overall patient satisfaction. A randomized group study by Du Plessis and colleagues[60] found that patients who received manual and manipulative therapy post–hallux valgus surgery had improved functional scores using the Foot Function Index, whereas those treated with only a night splint regressed when its use was discontinued. Studies are needed to determine the prevalence of physical therapy after hallux valgus correction and the efficacy of physical therapy at different time frames postoperatively. Nevertheless, based on this discussion, physical therapy should be strongly considered after hallux valgus correction (**Boxes 1** and **2**).

Box 1
Physical therapy evaluation tests and measures

- Pain
- Girth measurements
- Range of motion
- Muscle performance
- Joint mobility
- Soft tissue restrictions
- Gait evaluation
- Balance
- Neurosensory deficits
- Function

Box 2
Summary of physical therapy interventions

- Patient education
  - Scar care
  - Home program
  - Injury prevention
  - Home, community, and leisure reintegration
  - Activities of daily living
- Therapeutic exercise
  - Aerobic capacity/reconditioning
  - Balance, coordination, and agility training
  - Sensory retraining/adaptation
  - Flexibility exercises for range of motion, muscle lengthening, and stretching
  - Gait and locomotion training
  - Strength, power, and endurance training
- Manual therapy techniques
  - Manual lymphatic drainage
  - Soft tissue work
  - Joint mobilization/manipulation
  - Scar mobilization
- Supportive devices
  - Compression garments
  - Adaptive footwear
  - Orthotic devices
  - Taping
- Physical agents
  - Cryotherapy
  - Superficial heat
  - Ultrasound
  - Light therapy
- Electrical stimulation
  - TENS
  - Electrical muscle stimulation
  - Neuromuscular electrical stimulation

Adapted from American Physical Therapy Association. Guide to physical therapist practice. Second edition. American Physical Therapy Association. Phys Ther 2001;81(1):9–746.

REFERENCES

1. Nix S, Smith M, Vicenzino B. Prevalence of hallux valgus in the general population: a systematic review and meta-analysis. J Foot Ankle Res 2010;3:21.
2. Wülker N, Mittag F. The treatment of hallux valgus. Dtsch Arztebl Int 2012;109: 857–68.
3. Torkki M, Malmivaara A, Seitsalo S, et al. Hallux valgus: immediate operation versus 1 year of waiting with or without orthoses: a randomized controlled trial of 209 patients. Acta Orthop Scand 2003;74:209–15.
4. Myerson MS, Badekas A. Hypermobility of the first ray [abstract]. Foot Ankle Clin 2000;5:469–84.
5. APMA Website. Available at: http://www.apma.org/learn/FootHealth.cfm? ItemNumber=979. Accessed October 27, 2013.
6. AAOS Website. Available at: http://orthoinfo.aaos.org/topic.cfm?topic=a00140. Accessed October 27, 2013.
7. American Physical Therapy Association. Guide to physical therapist practice. Second edition. American Physical Therapy Association. Phys Ther 2001;81(1):9–746.
8. Bemis-Dougherty A. Practice matters: what is ICF? PT Magazine 2009;17(1): 44–6.
9. Kernozek T, Roehrs T, McGarvey S. Analysis of plantar loading parameters pre and post surgical intervention for hallux vargus [abstract]. Clin Biomech (Bristol, Avon) 1997;12:S18–9.
10. Kernozek TW, Sterriker SA. Chevron (Austin) distal metatarsal osteotomy for hallux valgus: comparison of pre- and post-surgical characteristics [abstract]. Foot Ankle Int 2002;23:503–8.
11. Dhukaram V, Hullin MG, Senthil Kumar C. The Mitchell and Scarf osteotomies for hallux vaglus correction: a retrospective, comparative analysis using plantar pressures [abstract]. J Foot Ankle Surg 2006;45:400–9.
12. Schuh R, Hofstaetter SG, Adams S. Rehabilitation after hallux valgus surgery: importance of physical therapy to restore weight bearing of the first ray during the stance phase. Phys Ther 2009;89:934–45.
13. Solis G, Saxby T. Incidence of DVT following surgery of the foot and ankle [abstract]. Foot Ankle Int 2002;23:411–4.
14. Nix S, Vicenzino B, Smith M. Foot pain and functional limitation in healthy adults with hallux valgus: a cross-sectional study. BMC Musculoskelet Disord 2012;13:197.
15. Schuh R, Adams S, Hofstaetter SG, et al. Plantar loading after chevron osteotomy combined with postoperative physical therapy [abstract]. Foot Ankle Int 2010;31:980–6.
16. Shamus J, Shamus E, Gugel RN, et al. The effect of sesamoid mobilization, flexor hallucis strengthening, and gait training on reducing pain and restoring function in individuals with hallux limitus: a clinical trial. J Orthop Sports Phys Ther 2004;34:368–76.
17. Budiman-Mak E, Conrad KJ, Roach KE. The foot function index: a measure of foot pain and disability. J Clin Epidemiol 1991;44:561–70.
18. Hayes KW. Manual for physical agents. 5th edition. Upper Saddle River (NJ): Prentice Hall, Inc; 2000.
19. Jang H, Lee H. Meta-analysis of pain relief effects by laser irradiation on joint areas. Photomed Laser Surg 2012;30:405–17.
20. Hajek V, Dussart C, Klack F, et al. Neuropathic complications after 157 procedures of continuous popliteal nerve block for hallux valgus surgery. A retrospective study [abstract]. Orthop Traumatol Surg Res 2012;98:327–33.

21. Ieong E, Afolayan J, Little N, et al. The incidence and natural history of forefoot scar pain following open hallux valgus surgery. Foot Ankle Spec 2013;6:271–4.
22. Parry I, Sen S, Palmieri T, et al. Nonsurgical scar management of the face: does early versus late intervention affect outcome [abstract]. J Burn Care Res 2013; 34(5):569–75.
23. Yun I, Yoo HS, Kim YO, et al. Improved scar appearance with combined use of silicone gel and vitamin C for Asian patients: a comparative case series [abstract]. Aesthetic Plast Surg 2013;37(6):1176–81.
24. O'Brien L, Jones DJ. Silicone gel sheeting for preventing and treating hypertrophic and keloid scars [abstract]. Cochrane Database Syst Rev 2013;(9):CD003826.
25. Min PK, Goo BL. 830 nm light-emitting diode low level light therapy (LED -LLLT) enhances wound healing: a preliminary study [abstract]. Laser Ther 2013;22(1): 43–9.
26. Mamalis AD, Lev-Tov H, Nguyen DH, et al. Laser and light-based treatment of Keloids- a review. J Eur Acad Dermatol Venereol 2013. http://dx.doi.org/10.1111/jdv.12253.
27. Tannenbaum M. Iodine iontophoresis in reducing scar tissue. Phys Ther 1980; 60:792.
28. Saro C, Jensen I, Lindgren U, et al. Quality-of-life outcome after hallux valgus surgery [abstract]. Qual Life Res 2007;16:731–8.
29. Chou YH, Yoo HS, Kim YO, et al. Case report: manual lymphatic drainage and kinesio taping in the secondary malignant breast cancer-related lymphedema in an arm with arteriovenous fistula for hemodialysis [abstract]. Am J Hosp Palliat Care 2013;30(5):503–6.
30. O'Brien JG, Chennubhotla SA, Chennubhotla RV. Treatment of edema. Am Fam Physician 2005;71(11):2111–7.
31. Threlkeld AJ. The effects of manual therapy on connective tissue. Phys Ther 1992;72(12):893–902.
32. Dimonte P, Light H. Pathomechanics, gait deviations, and treatment of the rheumatoid foot: a clinical report. Phys Ther 1982;62:1148–56.
33. Hromádka R, Barták V, Sosna A, et al. Release of the lateral structures of the first metatarsophalangeal joint during hallux valgus surgery [abstract]. Acta Chir Orthop Traumatol Cech 2012;79:222–7 [in Czech].
34. Stewart S, Ellis R, Heath M, et al. Ultrasonic evaluation of the abductor hallucis muscle in hallux valgus: a cross-sectional observational study. BMC Musculoskelet Disord 2013;14:45.
35. Nix S, Vicenzino B, Collins N, et al. Gait parameters associated with hallux valgus: a systematic review. J Foot Ankle Res 2013;6:9.
36. Arinci Incel N, Genc H, Erdem HR, et al. Muscle imbalance in hallux valgus: an electromyographic study [abstract]. Am J Phys Med Rehabil 2003;82:345–9.
37. Dykyj D. Pathologic anatomy of hallux abducto valgus [abstract]. Clin Podiatr Med Surg 1989;6:1–15.
38. Aseyo D, Nathan H. Hallux sesamoid bones. Anatomical observations with special reference to osteoarthritis and hallux valgus [abstract]. Int Orthop 1984;8: 67–73.
39. Ramdasss R, Meyr AJ. The multiplanar effect of first metatarsal osteotomy on sesamoid position [abstract]. J Foot Ankle Surg 2010;49:63–7.
40. Judge MS, LaPointe S, Yu GV, et al. The effect of hallux abducto valgus surgery on the sesamoid apparatus position [abstract]. J Am Podiatr Med Assoc 1999; 89:551–9.

41. Aggarwal A, Kumar S, Kumar R. Therapeutic management of the hallux rigidus [abstract]. Rehabil Res Pract 2012;2012:479046.
42. John MM, Kalish S, Perns SV, et al. Dynamic splinting for postoperative hallux limitus: a randomized, controlled trial. J Am Podiatr Med Assoc 2011;101:285–8.
43. Connor JC, Berk DM, Hotz MW. Effects of continuous passive motion following Austin bunionectomy. A prospective review [abstract]. J Am Podiatr Med Assoc 1995;85:744–8.
44. Perry J. Gait analysis: normal and pathological function. Thorofare (NJ): Slack Inc; 1992.
45. The Pathokinesiology Service & Physical Therapy Department, Rancho Los Amigos National Rehabilitation Center. Observational gait analysis handbook. Downey (CA): Los Amigos Research and Education Institute; 1996.
46. Ferris L, Sharkey NA, Smith TS, et al. Influence of extrinsic plantar flexors on forefoot loading during heel rise [abstract]. Foot Ankle Int 1996;16:464–73.
47. Jacob HA. Forces acting in the forefoot during normal gait—an estimate [abstract]. Clin Biomech 2001;16:783–92.
48. Hislop HJ, Avers D, Brown M. Daniels and Worthingham's muscle testing: techniques of manual examination and performance testing. 9th edition. St Louis (MO): Elsevier; 2014.
49. Norkin CC, White DJ. Measurement of joint motion. 4th edition. Philadelphia: F.A. Davis Company; 2009.
50. Khamis S, Yizhar Z. Effect of feet hyperpronation on pelvic alignment in a standing position [abstract]. Gait Posture 2007;25(1):127–34.
51. Menz HB, Lord SR. Foot pain impairs balance and functional ability in community-dwelling older people [abstract]. J Am Podiatr Med Assoc 2001; 91:222–9.
52. Hunt KJ, Hurwit D. Use of patient-reported outcome measures in foot and ankle research [abstract]. J Bone Joint Surg Am 2013;95:e118.
53. Martin RL, Irrgang JJ. A survey of self-reported outcome instruments for the foot and ankle. J Orthop Sports Phys Ther 2007;37(2):72–84.
54. Roukis TS. Nonunion after arthrodesis of the first metatarsal-phalangeal joint: a systematic review [abstract]. J Foot Ankle Surg 2011;50:710–3.
55. Hagedorn T, Dufour AB, Riskowski JL, et al. Foot disorders, foot posture and foot function: the Framingham foot study. PLoS One 2013;8(9):e74364.
56. Coughlin MJ, Jones CP. Hallux valgus: demographics, etiology, and radiographic assessment [abstract]. Foot Ankle Int 2007;28:759–77.
57. Glasoe W, Nuckley D, Ludewig P. Hallux valgus and the first metatarsal arch segment: a theoretical biomechanical perspective. Phys Ther 2010;90:110–20.
58. Glasoe WM, Phadke V, Pena FA, et al. An image-based gait simulation study of tarsal kinematics in women with hallux valgus. Phys Ther 2013;93:1–12.
59. Glasoe WM, Yack HJ, Saltzman CL. Anatomy and biomechanics of the first ray. Phys Ther 1999;79:854–9.
60. Du Plessis M, Zipfel B, Brantingham JW, et al. Manual and manipulative therapy compared to night splint for symptomatic and hallux abducto valgus: an exploratory randomized clinical trial [abstract]. Foot (Edinb) 2011;21:71–8.

Index

Note: Page numbers of article titles are in **boldface** type.

A

B

C

Clin Podiatr Med Surg 31 (2014) 323–328
http://dx.doi.org/10.1016/S0891-8422(14)00013-5
0891-8422/14/$ – see front matter © 2014 Elsevier Inc. All rights reserved.

podiatric.theclinics.com